CONCISE GUIDE TO

Group Psychotherapy

D0834936

American Psychiatric Press
CONCISE GUIDES

Robert E. Hales, M.D.
Series Editor

CONCISE GUIDE TO

Group Psychotherapy

Sophia Vinogradov, M.D.

Research Fellow in Psychiatry
Stanford University School of Medicine and
Palo Alto Veterans Administration Medical Center
Stanford, California

Irvin D. Yalom, M.D.

Professor of Psychiatry
Stanford University School of Medicine
Stanford, California

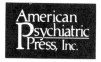

American
Psychiatric
Press, Inc.

1400 K Street, N.W.
Washington, DC 20005

First Edition   89 90 91   4 3 2 1

The paper used in this publication meets the minimum require-
ments of American National Standard for Information Sci-
ences—Permanence of Paper for Printed Library Materials,
ANSI Z39.48-1984.   ∞

Library of Congress Cataloging-in-Publication Data

Vinogradov, Sophia, 1958–
    Concise guide to group psychotherapy / Sophia Vinogradov, Irvin D. Yalom.
— 1st ed.
        p.   cm. — (Concise guides / American Psychiatric Press)
    Includes bibliographies.
    ISBN 0-88048-327-X (alk. paper)
    1. Group psychotherapy.   I. Yalom, Irvin D., 1931– .
    II. Title.   III. Series: Concise guides (American Psychiatric Press)
        [DNLM: 1. Psychotherapy, Group.   WM 430 V788c]
    RC488.V56   1989
    616.89′ 152—dc19
    DNLM/DLC
    for Library of Congress   88-38281
                                                             CIP

CONTENTS

INTRODUCTION

to the *American Psychiatric Press Concise Guides*

The *American Psychiatric Press Concise Guides* series provides, in a most accessible format, practical information for psychiatrists—and especially for psychiatry residents—working in such varied treatment settings as inpatient psychiatry services, outpatient clinics, consultation/liaison services, and private practice. The *Concise Guides* are meant to complement the more detailed information to be found in lengthier psychiatry texts.

The *Concise Guides* address topics of greatest concern to psychiatrists in clinical practice. The books in this series contain a detailed Table of Contents, along with an index, tables, and charts, for easy access; and their size, designed to fit into a lab coat pocket, makes them a convenient source of information. The number of references has been limited to those most relevant to the material presented.

The *Concise Guide to Group Psychotherapy* is written by two outstanding psychiatrists on the Stanford University Medical Center faculty: Drs. Sophia Vinogradov and Irvin D. Yalom. Dr. Vinogradov, one of the best and brightest of a new generation of psychiatrists, combines a solid background in basic research with excellent knowledge and experience in clinical psychiatry and group psychotherapy. Irvin D. Yalom is one of the greats of American psychiatry. His classic textbook, *The Theory and Practice of Group Psychotherapy,* is *the* standard against which all other volumes on group psychotherapy must be compared. Dr. Yalom has established himself as one of the country's leading experts in the field of group psychotherapy.

The two authors have complemented each other nicely in this *Guide.* Dr. Vinogradov, closer in time to her residency training, has presented practical and specific clinical pearls and techniques for psychiatry residents and other trainees to use in treating patients in group settings. Dr. Yalom's wisdom, extensive clinical experience, and unparalleled understanding of group psychotherapy theoretical issues are readily apparent throughout the book. By combining their respective talents and energies, they have produced a guide to group psychotherapy that will be read and reread both by residents who want to know the basics of this important treatment modality, and by more experienced psychiatrists and therapists who wish to refresh their knowledge.

The *Concise Guide to Group Psychotherapy* addresses the critical principles and techniques necessary to organize a group and conduct group psychotherapy. Chapter 1 defines group psychotherapy by summarizing its scope, clinical relevance, efficiency, and unique properties. Chapter 2 focuses on those therapeutic factors which contribute to the efficacy of group psychotherapy and emphasizes the forces that may influence these factors. Other chapters describe how to form a group, how to resolve common problems that occur in group therapy, and discuss important psychotherapeutic techniques that enhance group work. Finally, Drs. Vinogradov and Yalom discuss two specialized groups frequently formed in clinical practice: inpatient and outpatient groups.

Robert E. Hales, M.D.
Series Editor
American Psychiatric Press Concise Guides

ACKNOWLEDGMENTS

The authors wish to acknowledge Basic Books, Inc., publisher of *The Theory and Practice of Group Psychotherapy*, Third Edition, by Irvin D. Yalom (New York, Basic Books, 1985) and of *Inpatient Group Psychotherapy* by Irvin D. Yalom (New York, Basic Books, 1983). The large majority of the theoretical foundations and clinical concepts described in the present text are derived from these two works, and the reader is referred to them for a more detailed exposition of group psychotherapy.

Dr. Vinogradov gratefully acknowledges the help and support of Dr. Philippe M. Frossard in this and previous professional endeavors. She also thanks Dr. Mickey Indianer for discussions about substance abuse groups, and Dr. Serge N. Vinogradov and Dr. Terry Osback for their encouragement during the year prior to publication of this book.

WHAT IS GROUP PSYCHOTHERAPY?

Group psychotherapy is the application of psychotherapeutic techniques to a group of patients. But it is also something more. In individual psychotherapy, a trained person establishes a professional contract with a patient and makes verbal and nonverbal therapeutic interventions with the aim of alleviating psychological distress, changing maladaptive behavior, and encouraging personality growth and development.

In group therapy, however, both patient–patient interactions and patient–therapist interactions as they occur in the context of the group setting are used to effect changes in the maladaptive behavior of each of the group members. In other words, the group itself, as well as the application of specific techniques and interventions by the trained therapist, serves as a tool for change. This feature gives group psychotherapy its unique therapeutic potential.

■ THE SCOPE OF CURRENT GROUP PSYCHOTHERAPY PRACTICE

Today, group therapy encompasses a wide spectrum of practice which ranges from long-term interactional outpatient groups to acute crisis drop-in groups. This derives from three flexible characteristics of therapy groups: their setting, their goals, and their time frame (illustrated in Table 1).

CLINICAL SETTINGS

The clinical settings of psychotherapy groups vary widely and affect the entire structure and functioning of the group. Let us illustrate this point by comparing groups in two markedly different clinical settings: the psychiatric inpatient ward and the outpatient clinic.

Inpatient groups:
- take place on a psychiatric unit
- meet daily

TABLE 1. **The Range of Current Group Psychotherapy Practice**

Settings	Example of Group	Goals	Time Frame
Inpatient			
Acute inpatient psychiatric unit	Daily high-functioning level group	Restoration of function	1–2 days to several weeks
Chronic inpatient facility	Daily low-functioning small group	Rehabilitation	Weeks to months
Outpatient			
Private practice or general psychiatric clinic	Weekly interactional group	Symptom relief and character change	1–2 years
Psychiatric medication clinic	Monthly medication clinic drop-in group	Education; maintenance of function	Indefinite
Behavioral medicine clinic group	Weekly eating disorders	Discrete behavior change	2–3 months
Substance abuse treatment center	Daily early alcohol recovery group	Confrontation of denial; maintenance of sobriety	3 months
Specialized medical clinic	Diabetes support group	Education; support; socialization	Indefinite
Counseling center	Weekly bereavement group	Support; catharsis; socialization	2–3 months

- are composed of individuals with various acute psychiatric problems
- are mandatory
- have rapid turnover in group membership because of the short duration of hospitalization.

Outpatient groups:
- are voluntary groups with stable membership
- meet once weekly in a psychiatric clinic
- consist of individuals who show similar and stable levels of functioning.

There are exceptions to this simple dichotomy. Some inpatient wards form homogeneous voluntary groups based on level of functioning, although their membership still shifts a great deal from day to day. And psychiatric outpatient groups encompass many variations, ranging from the monthly drop-in group held for chronically ill patients in a medication clinic to the twice-weekly interactional group run in a private practitioner's office.

Inpatient versus outpatient is one distinction in a range of settings, but group therapy is also practiced in myriad other clinical situations. These extend from the daily small groups held in a psychiatric day hospital to weekly probation groups to staff retreats or support groups. Specialized groups for medical syndromes, such as diabetes education groups or lupus support groups, are often held in a hospital or outpatient setting, while other types of specialized groups—rape crisis groups, Vietnam veterans groups—are associated with centers that offer specific kinds of counseling services, such as a rape trauma center, or a veterans outreach center.

GOALS

The goals of psychotherapy groups occupy a wide spectrum. At one end are found the ambitious goals of long-term interactional groups: symptom relief and character change. At the other end is the more limited but crucial goal of restoration of function and preparation for discharge, such as may occur in acute inpatient therapy groups.

Between these two extremes lie the therapeutic goals of the large majority of psychotherapy groups. For some, such as medication clinic groups or in- and outpatient groups for the chronic mentally ill, the most important goal is maintenance of appropriate psychosocial functioning. Many others, including social skills training groups and specialized and self-help groups, provide education, socialization, and support. Most symptom-oriented short-term groups which are behaviorally focused (for example, those aimed at bulimia, agoraphobia, or smoking cessation) have the goals of discrete behavior change.

TIME FRAMES

The time frame of a psychotherapy group consists of the life of the group (the number of sessions it will meet) and the length of stay of group members. Both of these factors are intertwined with the clinical setting and goals of the group; both vary widely. Inpatient groups, for example, are an indelible part of the treatment program and are thus indefinitely self-sustaining; the ward census may change, different kinds of patients may or may not be hospitalized, but the group is held every day, rain or shine. The life of an outpatient group is much more variable. Outpatient groups can exist for one session only—say, a drop-in crisis group held as needed at a student health center—or can be open-ended and long-term in nature, periodically renewing their membership as patients graduate and are replaced by new members.

The length of stay of group members depends on the goals of the group. In an interactionally oriented outpatient group with ambitious clinical goals, members obtain maximum therapeutic benefit after one to three years. The life of the group is indefinite and graduating members are replaced as they leave in order to keep the group size approximately constant. But other types of groups in the outpatient setting use a time-limited format, especially if they are focusing on a specific problem. For example, an educational-behavioral group for patients with eating disorders may be designed to meet for 12 sessions. The issues addressed in this kind of a group and the manner in which they are addressed will of necessity be very different from those of the long-term group.

■ THE CLINICAL RELEVANCE OF GROUP PSYCHOTHERAPY

Although the scope of current group psychotherapy practice is far-ranging, mainstream psychiatric education has de-emphasized the teaching and practice of group psychotherapy in recent years. The remedicalization of psychiatry, with its interest in biological causes and pharmacological treatments for mental illness, may account for this trend. Nonetheless, group therapy is a widely practiced mode of treatment employed in a vast number of settings with a proven degree of effectiveness.

CLINICAL EFFICACY

Group psychotherapy is effective treatment, at least as effective as individual psychotherapy in treating various psychological disorders (1). Thirty-two studies which directly contrasted individual and group treatments for interpersonal problems were analyzed (2). In 24 of the studies, there were no significant differences between the two modalities. In the remaining eight, group psychotherapy was found to be more effective than individual psychotherapy.

Multiple outcome studies have tested the efficacy of group treatment for a wide range of psychological problems and behavioral disorders ranging from neurotic interpersonal behavior to sociopathy, substance abuse, and chronic mental illness (3–5). This large body of research evidence supports the widespread clinical consensus that group psychotherapy is beneficial to its participants.

TREATMENT POPULATIONS

Enormous numbers of psychiatric patients receive their sole or primary treatment in groups. This is particularly true in institutional settings and in the treatment of the chronic mentally ill. At least one-half of all psychiatric hospitals and one-quarter of all correctional institutions, not to mention the vast majority of community mental health centers, use group treatments (6). Many health maintenance organizations (HMOs) make substantial use of group therapy as well (7). Altogether, this represents a potential patient population in the hundreds of thousands.

NONPSYCHIATRIC GROUPS

Vast numbers of nonpsychiatric patients attend specialized treatment groups. The use of education and support groups for family members and for individuals with chronic illness or with particular medical conditions is burgeoning in the health-care setting. Diabetes education groups, groups for spouses coping with Alzheimer's disease, cancer support groups, and post-myocardial infarction rehabilitation groups are just a few examples of a growing mode of psychosocial intervention.

Self-help groups and self-awareness groups are yet another form of treatment and intervention used by large numbers of nonpsychiatric clients. Perhaps 12 to 14 million individuals attended some form of self-help group in 1983, groups such as Alcoholics Anonymous, Compassionate Friends, and Recovery, Inc. (8). Hundreds of thousands of Americans continue to seek involvement in large group awareness training represented by enterprises such as est or Lifespring. The corporate world routinely uses seminars and retreats which harness the principles of group dynamics in order to strengthen the management skills of top executives. Inevitably, the practicing therapist of nearly every persuasion will encounter patients who have had prior contact with some form of group experience.

■ EFFICIENCY OF GROUP PSYCHOTHERAPY

The fact that group treatment is employed with such a large number of patients and clients is indicative of its efficiency as a mode of psychotherapeutic intervention.

EFFICIENT USE OF RESOURCES

To facilitate the treatment of large numbers of tuberculosis patients, a turn-of-the-century Boston internist named Joseph Pratt used group meetings to educate and treat his patients. Many of his patients were indigent and could not afford private care; many were debilitated, despondent, and ostracized from the healthy community. Pratt organized groups of 20 or 30 patients and lectured them once or twice a week (9); this marked the beginning of group therapy.

Today, group therapy still retains this advantageous feature of expediency. Large numbers of patients can be treated with efficient use of time, space, personnel, and other resources. In community agencies and institutional settings, where huge caseloads of patients must be seen by a limited number of health care workers, a group meeting permits useful psychotherapy to take place even when the staff-to-patient ratio is too low to allow it to occur on an individual basis.

COST-EFFECTIVENESS

Pratt worked with indigent patients too poor to pay for alternative treatment, and several other early pioneers in the group-lecture approach treated psychotic individuals who could afford only institutional care. In England during and after World War II, the overwhelming number of psychiatric casualties and the limited number of hospital staff and economic resources made group treatment the most practical modality available—and led to an explosion in group therapy practice and research.

Group treatment has been shown in at least one study to be more consistently efficient and/or cost-effective than individual treatment (2). In a future where third-party payers loom large, these practical considerations of expediency and cost-effectiveness will become more influential. More than one prescient group therapist has suggested that soon clinicians will need to justify individual therapy, and defend their decision not to use the more cost-effective group therapy! (10).

■ UNIQUE PROPERTIES OF GROUP PSYCHOTHERAPY

Although group therapy is more cost-effective, its advantages transcend simple economic considerations: It is a form of treatment that makes use of unique therapeutic properties not shared by other psychotherapies. Group therapy is an unparalleled mode of psychotherapy because it relies upon a very powerful therapeutic tool, the group setting. The power of this tool derives from the importance that interpersonal interactions play in our psychological development.

INTERPERSONAL RELATIONSHIPS AND PSYCHOLOGICAL DEVELOPMENT

In describing the Wild Child of Aveyron in 1799, a French psychologist noted that to raise a child completely separate from human society and human interactions resulted in "a state of vacuity and barbarism ... a state in which the individual, deprived of the characteristic faculties of his species, drags on miserably, equally without intelligence and without affections ... " (11). A full complement of interpersonal relationships is crucially important to normal human psychological development.

Following this simple premise, personality and patterns of behavior can be seen as the result of early interactions with other significant human beings. We know, for example, that successful attachment and bonding are imperative for adaptive psychological development in both primates and in humans. Harry Stack Sullivan was one of the first psychiatrists and theorists to underscore the link between psychopathology and a developmental history of distorted interpersonal relationships (12). Modern schools of dynamic psychotherapy emphasize that psychiatric treatment must be directed toward understanding and correcting these interpersonal distortions.

GROUP PSYCHOTHERAPY PROVIDES INTERPERSONAL INTERACTIONS

If we agree with Sullivan's contention that the personality is almost entirely the product of interaction with other significant human beings, and that psychopathology arises when these interactions and their attendant perceptions and expectations are distorted, then it follows that psychiatric treatment should be directed toward the correction of interpersonal distortions. The goal of this kind of treatment is very specific: to enable the individual to participate collaboratively with others and to obtain interpersonal satisfactions in the context of realistic, mutually gratifying relationships—in sum, to lead a more abundant and rewarding life with others (13). "One achieves mental health to the extent that one becomes aware of one's interpersonal relationships" (14).

Although the examination and correction of interpersonal distortions can take place in the context of a two-person, therapist–patient relationship, a group of several people meeting together provides a larger and potentially more powerful interpersonal arena. In the group setting, patients are provided with a varied array of relationships; they must interact with each other, with the group leaders, with people from differing backgrounds, with same-sex members and with members of the opposite sex. Members must learn to deal with their likes, dislikes, similarities, dissimilarities, envy, timidity, aggression, fear, attraction, and competitiveness. This all takes place under the scrutiny of the group where, with careful therapeutic leadership, members give and obtain feedback about the meaning and effect of their various interactions on each other. In this way, the group setting itself becomes an immensely specific therapeutic tool.

COHESIVE GROUP EXPERIENCES

The potential power of group therapy derives also from a curious phenomenon reported in many segments of our society: a pervasive sense of increasing interpersonal and social isolation. Group experiences themselves are ubiquitous, but cohesive, supportive, self-reflective group experiences seem to be more and more elusive in our modern, industrialized lives. Groups are an integral part of our developmental experiences, from our early family unit, to the classroom, to the people we surround ourselves with at work, at play, and at home. At the same time, we hear complaints about increasing interpersonal alienation in modern life, a sense of isolation, anonymity, and social fragmentation.

Perhaps because of this, and because it can provide such a powerful and unique therapeutic experience, the group setting is being used more and more, not only by mental health professionals but by laymen. Myriad specialized groups function in a supportive and occasionally highly therapeutic mode, and the examples are legion. Alcoholics Anonymous, Parents without Partners, Recovery, Inc. (for coping with emotional stress), Overeaters Anonymous, and Mended Hearts (for patients who have survived myocardial infarction) are but a few of the current specialized and self-help groups available in the lay setting. The burgeoning number of groups being used in settings that are nonpsychiatric indicates a general need among the lay public for cohesive, supportive group experiences.

■ REFERENCES

1. Smith M, Glass G, Miller T: The Benefits of Psychotherapy. Baltimore, Johns Hopkins University Press, 1980
2. Toseland RW, Siporin M: When to recommend group treatment: a review of the clinical and the research literature. Int J Group Psychother 1986; 32:171-201
3. Bednar RL, Lawlis GF: Empirical research on group psychotherapy, in Handbook of Psychotherapy and Behavior Change, 2nd ed. Edited by Bergin AE, Garfield S. New York, Wiley, 1971
4. Parloff MB, Dies RR: Group psychotherapy outcome research 1966-1975. Int J Group Psychother 1977; 27:281-319
5. Kanas N: Group therapy with schizophrenics: a review of controlled studies. Int J Group Psychother 1986; 36:339-351
6. Shapiro DA, Shapiro D: Meta-analysis of comparative therapy outcome studies: a replication and refinement. Psychol Bull 1982; 92:581-604
7. Cheifetz DI, Salloway JC: Patterns of mental health services provided by HMOs. Am Psychol 1984; 39:495-502
8. Lieberman M: Self-help groups and psychiatry, in Psychiatry Update: American Psychiatric Association Annual Review, vol. 5. Edited by Frances AJ, Hales RE. Washington, DC, American Psychiatric Press, 1986
9. Pratt JH: The principles of class treatment and their application to various chronic diseases. Hospital Social Service 1922; 6:404
10. Dies RR: Practical, theoretical and empirical foundations for group psychotherapy, in Psychiatry Update: American Psychiatric Association Annual Review, vol. 5. Edited by Frances AJ, Hales RE. Washington, DC, American Psychiatric Press, 1986
11. Malson L: Wolf Children and the Problem of Human Nature. New York, Monthly Review Press, 1972
12. Sullivan HS: The Interpersonal Theory of Psychiatry. New York, W.W. Norton, 1953
13. Yalom ID: The Theory and Practice of Group Psychotherapy, 3rd ed. New York, Basic Books, 1985
14. Sullivan HS: Conceptions of Modern Psychiatry. New York, W.W. Norton, 1940

WHAT MAKES GROUP PSYCHOTHERAPY WORK? 2

Group psychotherapy makes use of specific therapeutic factors. We must identify these specific factors if we are to understand the common ways in which vastly different kinds of groups help members to change. Such a simplifying principle helps us also to understand what happens to different members within the same group.

■ THE THERAPEUTIC FACTORS

Over the past three decades, a variety of research approaches have been used to answer the question, "What makes group psychotherapy work?"—including the interview and testing of group therapy patients with successful outcomes, as well as questionnaires directed at experienced group therapists and trained observers. From these methods, researchers have identified a number of mechanisms of change in group psychotherapy: the curative or therapeutic factors (1).

There is a high degree of overlap among the various classification systems proposed by different investigators (2–4). Yalom has developed an empirically based, 11-factor inventory of the therapeutic mechanisms operating in group psychotherapy, as follows:

1. Instillation of hope
2. Universality
3. Imparting of information
4. Altruism
5. Development of socializing techniques
6. Imitative behavior
7. Catharsis
8. Corrective recapitulation of the primary family group
9. Existential factors
10. Group cohesiveness
11. Interpersonal learning

INSTILLATION OF HOPE

Faith in a treatment mode is itself therapeutically effective, both when the patient has a high expectation of help and when the therapist believes in the efficacy of the treatment (5, 6). Although the instillation and maintenance of hope are crucial to all of the psychotherapies, this plays a unique role in the group setting.

In every therapy group, there are patients who have improved as well as members who are at a low ebb. Patients often remark at the end of therapy that to have observed the improvement of others offered them great hope for their own improvement. Groups such as Alcoholics Anonymous, which are aimed at alcohol and substance abusers, use the testimonials of ex-alcoholics or recovered addicts to inspire hope in new members. Many of the self-help groups that have emerged in the past decade, such as Compassionate Friends (for bereaved parents) or Mended Heart (for cardiac surgery patients), also place a heavy emphasis on the instillation of hope.

UNIVERSALITY

Many patients go through life with an overwhelming sense of isolation. They are secretly convinced that they are unique in their loneliness or their wretchedness, that they alone have certain unacceptable problems or impulses. Such people are often socially isolated and have few opportunities for frank and candid social interchange. In a therapy group, especially in its early stages, patients experience a powerful sense of relief when they realize they are not alone with their problems.

Some specialized groups, in fact, are focused on helping individuals for whom secrecy has been an especially important and isolating part of life. For example, many short-term structured groups for bulimic patients require open disclosure about attitudes toward body image and detailed accounts about bingeing and purging behavior. As a rule, patients experience great relief as they discover that they are not alone, and that their problems are universal and are shared by other group members.

IMPARTING INFORMATION

The imparting of information occurs in a group whenever a therapist gives didactic instruction to patients about mental or physical functioning, or whenever advice or direct guidance about life problems is offered either by the leader or by other group members. Although long-term interactional groups generally do not value the use of didactic education or advice, other types of groups rely more heavily on advice or instruction.

DIDACTIC INSTRUCTION

Many self-help groups—such as Alcoholics Anonymous, Recovery, Inc., Make Today Count (for cancer patients), Gamblers Anonymous, and the like—emphasize didactic instruction. A text is used, experts are invited to address the group, and members are strongly encouraged to exchange information. Specialized groups aimed at patients with a specific medical or psychological disorder or facing a specific life crisis (for example, obese individuals, rape victims, epileptics, chronic pain patients) build in a didactic component; leaders offer explicit instruction about the nature of the individual's illness or life situation. Therapists leading specialized groups often teach members ways of developing coping mechanisms and implementing stress-reduction or relaxation techniques.

ADVICE-GIVING

Unlike explicit didactic instruction from the therapist, direct advice from the members occurs without exception in every kind of therapy group. Noninteractionally focused groups make explicit and effective use of direct suggestions and guidance from both the leader and other members. For example, behavior-shaping groups, discharge groups (preparing patients for discharge from the hospital), Recovery, Inc., and Alcoholics Anonymous all proffer considerable direct advice. Discharge groups may discuss the events of a patient's trial home visit and offer suggestions for alternative behavior, while Alcoholics Anonymous and Recovery, Inc. use guidance and directive slogans ("One day at a time" or "Ninety meetings in ninety days"). Research on a behavior-shaping group of male sex offenders noted that the most effective form of guidance was through systematic operationalized instructions or through alternative suggestions about how to reach a desired goal (7).

In dynamic interactional therapy groups, advice-giving invariably is part of the early life of the group, but is of limited value to the members. Later, when the group as a whole has moved beyond the problem-solving stage and has begun to engage in interactional work, the reappearance of advice-seeking or advice-giving around a given issue suggests that the group is avoiding the work of therapy.

ALTRUISM

In every therapy group, patients become enormously helpful to one another: They share similar problems and they offer each other support, reassurance, suggestions, and insight. To the patient starting therapy who is demoralized and who feels that he or she has nothing of value to offer anyone, the experience of being helpful to other members of the group can be surprisingly rewarding, and is one of the reasons that group therapy so often boosts self-esteem. The therapeutic factor of altruism is unique to group therapy; patients in individual psychotherapy almost never have the experience of being helpful to their psychotherapist.

The altruistic act not only boosts self-esteem, it also distracts patients who spend much of their psychic energy immersed in morbid self-absorption. The patient caught up in ruminations about his or her own psychological woes is suddenly forced to be helpful to someone else. By its very structure, the therapy group fosters the act of aiding others and counters solipsism.

DEVELOPMENT OF SOCIALIZING TECHNIQUES

Social learning—the development of basic social skills— is a therapeutic factor that operates in all psychotherapy groups, although the nature of the skills taught and the explicitness of the process vary greatly depending upon the type of group. In some groups, such as those preparing long-term hospitalized patients for discharge or those for adolescents with behavioral problems, there is explicit emphasis on the development of social skills. Role playing techniques are often used to prepare patients for job interviews or to teach adolescent boys how to invite a girl to a dance.

In groups that are more interactionally oriented, patients learn about maladaptive social behavior from the honest feedback they offer each other. A patient may, for example, learn about a disconcerting tendency to avoid eye contact during conversation, or about the effect that his or her whispery voice and constantly folded arms has on others, or about a host of other habits which, unbeknownst to the patient, have been undermining his or her social relationships.

IMITATIVE BEHAVIOR

The importance of imitative behavior as a therapeutic factor is difficult to gauge, but social psychological research indicates that psychotherapists underestimate its importance (8). In group therapy, members benefit from observing the therapy of another patient with similar problems, a phenomenon referred to as vicarious learning.

For example, a timid, repressed female member who observes another woman in the group experiment with more extroverted behavior and a more attractive appearance may then, herself, similarly experiment with new methods of grooming and self-presentation. Or an emotionally restricted, lonely male member may begin to imitate another man in the group who has received positive feedback from women members by expressing himself openly and frankly.

CATHARSIS

Catharsis, or the ventilation of emotions, is a complex therapeutic factor that is linked to other processes in a group, particularly universality and cohesiveness. The sheer act of ventilation, by itself, although accompanied by a sense of emotional relief, rarely promotes lasting change for a patient. It is the affective sharing of one's inner world, and then the acceptance by others in the group, that is of paramount importance. To be able to express strong and deep emotions, and yet still be accepted by others, brings into question one's belief that one is basically repugnant, unacceptable, or unlovable.

Psychotherapy is both an emotional and a corrective experience. In order for change to take place, a patient must first experience something strongly in the group setting and undergo the sense of catharsis accompanying that strong emotional experience. Then the patient must proceed to integrate the cathartic event by understanding the meaning of the event, first, in the context of the group, and second, in the context of his or her outside life. This principle is discussed further in the section on interpersonal learning and the here-and-now focus of group psychotherapy.

CORRECTIVE RECAPITULATION OF THE PRIMARY FAMILY GROUP

Many patients enter group therapy with a history of highly unsatisfactory experiences in their first and most important group: the primary family. Because group therapy offers such a vast array of recapitulative possibilities, patients may begin to interact with leaders or other members as they once interacted with parents and siblings.

A helplessly dependent patient may imbue the leader with unrealistic knowledge and power. A rebellious and defiant individual may regard the therapist as someone who blocks autonomy in the group or who strips members of their individuality. The primitive or chaotic patient might attempt to split the cotherapists or even the entire group, igniting fires of bitter disagreement. The competitive patient will compete with other members for the therapist's attention, or perhaps seek allies in an effort to topple the therapists. And a self-effacing individual may neglect his or her own interests in a seemingly selfless effort to placate or provide for other members. All of these patterns of behavior can represent a recapitulation of early family experiences.

What is of capital importance in interactional group psychotherapy (and to a lesser degree in other group settings that make use of psychological insight) is not only that these kinds of early familial conflicts are re-enacted, but that they are recapitulated correctively. The group leader must not permit these growth-inhibiting relationships to freeze into the rigid, impenetrable system that characterizes many family structures. Instead, the leader must explore and challenge fixed roles in the group, and continually encourage members to test new behaviors.

EXISTENTIAL FACTORS

An existential approach to the understanding of patients' problems posits that the human being's paramount struggle is with the givens of our existence: death, isolation, freedom, and meaninglessness (9). In certain kinds of psychotherapy groups, particularly those centered around patients with cancer or chronic and life-threatening medical illnesses, or in bereavement groups, these existential givens play a central role in therapy.

Even standard therapy groups have considerable traffic with existential concerns if the group leader is informed and sensitive to these issues. In the course of therapy, members begin to realize that there is a limit to the guidance and support they can receive from others. They may find that the ultimate responsibility for the autonomy of the group and for the conduct of their lives is their own. They learn that, although one can be close to others, there is nonetheless a basic aloneness to existence that cannot be avoided. As they accept some of these issues, they learn to face their limitations with greater candor and courage. In group psychotherapy, the sound and trusting relationship among the members—the basic, intimate encounter—has an intrinsic value as it provides presence and a "being with" in the face of these harsh existential realities.

COHESIVENESS

Group cohesiveness is one of the more complex and absolutely integral features of a successful psychotherapy group. Group cohesiveness refers to the attractiveness that members have for their group and for the other members. The members of a cohesive group are accepting of one another, supportive, and inclined to form meaningful relationships in the group. Research indicates that cohesive groups achieve better therapeutic outcomes (10).

Just as, in individual psychotherapy, it is the relationship itself between therapist and patient that heals, cohesiveness is the group therapy analog of this therapist–patient relationship. Most psychiatric patients have had an impoverished history of belonging—never before have they been a valuable, integral, participating member of any kind of group, and the sheer successful negotiation of a group therapy experience is, in itself, curative. Furthermore, the social behavior required for members to be esteemed by a cohesive group is also adaptive to the individual in his or her social life outside of the group.

Group cohesiveness also provides conditions of acceptance and understanding. Patients are, under cohesive conditions, more inclined to express and explore themselves, to become aware of and integrate hitherto unacceptable aspects of themselves, and to relate more deeply to others. Cohesiveness in a group favors self-disclosure, risk-taking, and the constructive expression of confrontation and conflict, all phenomena that facilitate successful psychotherapy.

Highly cohesive groups are stable groups with better attendance, active patient commitment and participation, and minimal membership turnover. Some group settings, such as those specializing in a particular problem or disorder (a cancer support group, a group for women law students run by a university health center) will, because of the members' shared problems, develop a great deal of immediate cohesiveness. In other kinds of groups, especially those where membership changes frequently, the leader must actively facilitate the development of this important and pervasive therapeutic factor (see Chapter 7).

■ INTERPERSONAL LEARNING: A COMPLEX AND POWERFUL THERAPEUTIC FACTOR

In group psychotherapy, each member is provided, ready-made, with a unique ensemble of interpersonal interactions to explore. Yet the potent therapeutic factor of interpersonal learning is often overlooked, misapplied, or misunderstood by leaders, perhaps because the understanding and encouragement of interpersonal exploration requires considerable therapist skill and experience. In order to define and understand the use of interpersonal learning in group therapy, we must examine four underlying concepts:

1. The importance of interpersonal relationships
2. The necessity of corrective emotional experiences for successful psychotherapy
3. The group as a social microcosm
4. Learning from behavioral patterns in the social microcosm

THE IMPORTANCE OF INTERPERSONAL RELATIONSHIPS

Interpersonal relationships contribute not only to the development of personality, as we discussed earlier, but to the genesis of psychopathology. Interpersonal interactions can thus be used in therapy both to understand and to treat psychological disturbances.

INTERPERSONAL RELATIONSHIPS AND THE DEVELOPMENT OF PSYCHOPATHOLOGY

Given the prolonged period of helplessness during infancy, the need for interpersonal acceptance and security is as crucial to the survival of the developing child as any basic biological need (11). To ensure and promote this interpersonal acceptance, a developing child accentuates those aspects of his or her behavior that meet with approval or obtain desired ends, and suppresses those aspects that engender punishment or disapproval. The little girl who grows up in a rigid household where the expression of emotion is discouraged, for example, soon learns to squelch her spontaneous feelings in favor of more detached behavior.

Psychopathology arises when interactions with significant others have resulted in fixed distortions that persist into life beyond the period of original shaping—distortions in how one tends to perceive others, distortions in the understanding of one's own needs and the needs of others, distortions in how one reacts to various interpersonal interactions. "There seems to be no agent more effective than another person in bringing a world for oneself alive, or, by a glance, a gesture, or a remark, shriveling up the reality in which one is lodged." (12)

INTERPERSONAL RELATIONSHIPS AND PRESENTING SYMPTOMS

Patients are generally unaware of the importance of interpersonal issues in their clinical condition. They seek treatment for the alleviation of various troubling symptoms, such as anxiety or depression. The first task of the interpersonally oriented psychotherapist is to concentrate upon the interpersonal pathology which underlies a particular symptom complex; in other words, the therapist translates psychological or psychiatric symptoms into interpersonal language.

Consider, for example, the patient who complains of depression. It is rarely fruitful for the psychotherapist to address "depression" per se. The typical symptom cluster of dysphoric mood and neurovegetative signs does not in and of itself offer a handhold to begin the process of psychotherapeutic change. Instead, the therapist relates to the person who is depressed and ascertains the underlying interpersonal problems that both arise from and exacerbate the depression (problems such as dependency, obsequiousness, inability to express rage, and hypersensitivity to rejection).

Once these maladaptive interpersonal themes have been identified, the therapist has more tangible issues to address. Dependency, rage, obsequiousness, and hypersensitivity will all emerge in the therapeutic relationship and will be accessible to analysis and to change.

CORRECTIVE EMOTIONAL EXPERIENCES

Therapy is an emotional and a corrective experience. Patients must experience something strongly, but they must also understand the implications of that emotional experience. Therapeutic work consists of an alternating sequence of, first, affect evocation and expression, and second, the analysis and understanding of that affect. Franz Alexander introduced the concept of the "corrective emotional experience" in 1946: "The patient, in order to be helped, must undergo a corrective emotional experience suitable to repair the traumatic influence of previous experience (13)."

These two basic principles of individual psychotherapy—the importance of a strong emotional experience and the patient's discovery that his or her reactions are inappropriate—are equally crucial to group psychotherapy. In fact, the group setting offers far more opportunities for the genesis of corrective emotional experiences, as it contains a host of built-in tensions and multiple interpersonal situations to which the patient must react.

For the interactions inherent in a group setting to be translated into corrective emotional experiences, two fundamental conditions are required:

1. The members must experience the group as sufficiently safe and supportive so that they are willing to express basic differences and tensions.
2. There must be sufficient feedback and honesty of expression to permit effective reality testing.

The corrective emotional experience in group psychotherapy thus has several components, summarized in Table 1.

THE GROUP AS SOCIAL MICROCOSM

A corrective emotional experience can occur in a group when basic tensions and modes of relating are allowed to emerge in a safe and honest environment, followed by examination of (and learning from) the ensuing interpersonal interactions. What makes group psychotherapy an ideal arena for this kind of interpersonal learning is that individual group members create their characteristic interactional tensions and engage in their maladaptive modes of relating to others right there in the group setting. Put another way, the therapy group becomes a social microcosm for each of its members, a microcosm in which each member can then undergo corrective emotional experiences.

TABLE 1. Components of the Corrective Emotional Experience in Group Psychotherapy

Features of Group	Process	Result
Safe environment Supportive interactions	Expression of basic tensions and emotions	Affect evocation
Open feedback Honest reactions	Reality testing and examination of each member's emotional experience	Affect integration

DEVELOPMENT OF THE SOCIAL MICROCOSM

Sooner or later (given enough time and freedom, and provided that the group is experienced as safe), each member's underlying interpersonal tensions and distortions begin to emerge. Each person in the group begins to interact with other group members in the same way that he or she interacts with people outside of the group. Patients create in the group the same type of interpersonal world they inhabit on the outside. Competition for attention, struggles for dominance and status, sexual tensions, stereotyped distortions about background and values, all come to light.

The group becomes a laboratory experiment in which interpersonal strengths and weaknesses unfold in miniature. Slowly, but predictably, each individual's interpersonal pathology is displayed before the other group members. Arrogance, impatience, narcissism, grandiosity, sexualization—all such traits eventually surface and become enacted in the confines of the group.

In a group that is encouraged to free-run in a safe, interactionally oriented manner, there is almost no need for members to describe their past or to report present difficulties with relationships in their outside life. As in the clinical vignettes below, patients' group behavior provides far more accurate and immediate data. Individual members begin to act out their specific interpersonal problems before the eyes of everyone in the group and perpetuate their distortions under the collective scrutiny of fellow members. A freely interacting group eventually develops into a social microcosm of each of the members of that group.

CLINICAL VIGNETTES

Elizabeth was an attractive woman who, after her husband's job promotion and transfer, had left a high-powered career and had a baby; she soon entered a severe depression, and felt overwhelmed by pain she couldn't express. She found her life lacking in intimacy, and her outside relationships, including her marriage, felt superficial and unauthentic. In the group, Elizabeth was very popular. She was charming, sensitive, and concerned about everyone. However, she rarely let the group see behind her composed facade and into the depths of her pain and despair. Her great shame about her depression (after all, she was wealthy, privileged, and "had it so good") and even deeper shame about the childhood of poverty and abuse from which she had risen resulted in her recreating in the group the same type of cordial but distant and unnourishing relationships she had established in her social life and marriage.

Alan joined the group complaining that his life contained no emotional highs or lows, but just a neutral, functional evenness. He had no close friends, and although he was extremely successful professionally, he had a compulsive, competitive, and intimidating attitude in the workplace that kept colleagues at a distance. Although he dated frequently, the thrill of the initial sexual conquest would inevitably pall; a woman he was most interested in had refused to commit to a relationship with him and had left the area, leaving him with a feeling of emptiness. Alan soon recreated this situation in miniature in the therapy group. Although he was an active and articulate member, he devoted himself to establishing a witty but condescending dominance over the women in the group, including the female cotherapist. The female members began to feel belittled and withdrew from him. He also adopted an exceedingly competitive and intimidating stance with the men in the group, and soon all the members began avoiding any meaningful or emotionally-laden interactions with him. Alan quickly succeeded in isolating himself from all fulfilling relationships in the social microcosm of the group, perpetuating his pervasive feeling of emptiness.

Bob was a young, rebellious artist with a delinquent tinge. His outside life was characterized by defiance toward authority and professional status, a defiance that was puerile and ineffective rather than the result of mature assertiveness. He eschewed real competition in his social and work life, and this attitude was seriously hampering his financial and professional success. In the group, he quickly adopted the role of provocateur, and he frequently challenged and prodded members. His relationship with the male cotherapist became especially complex: Bob soon found himself unable to look at the therapist face-to-face, or accept any positive feedback from him. When questioned, Bob would refuse to respond, and at times said he was afraid he would start to cry. This group work began to clarify the other side of Bob's defiance, and gradually he began to understand the counterdependent nature of his rebelliousness: Bob in fact had many dependent yearnings and a strong desire to be cared for, and his fear of those cravings led him to adopt his characteristic defiant attitude both in the group and in his life outside the group.

LEARNING FROM BEHAVIOR IN THE SOCIAL MICROCOSM

Because of the wide range of corrective emotional experiences offered in the group setting, the process of group psychotherapy provides the therapist with an extremely powerful tool for change, that of interpersonal learning. This process—in which psychopathology emerges from and is embodied in distorted interpersonal interactions; in which the group becomes a social microcosm as each member displays his or her interpersonal pathology; and in which feedback allows each member to experience, to identify, and to change his or her maladaptive interpersonal behavior—is schematically outlined in the following sequence and summarized in Table 2 (14, 15):

1. Psychopathology and symptomatology emerge from and are perpetuated by maladaptive interpersonal relationships; many of these maladaptive interpersonal relationships are based on distortions that arise from early developmental experiences.

TABLE 2. **Learning from Behavioral Patterns in the Social Microcosm of the Group**

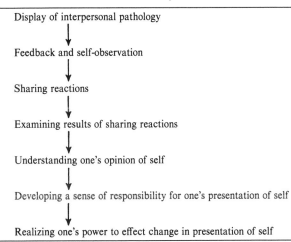

Display of interpersonal pathology

↓

Feedback and self-observation

↓

Sharing reactions

↓

Examining results of sharing reactions

↓

Understanding one's opinion of self

↓

Developing a sense of responsibility for one's presentation of self

↓

Realizing one's power to effect change in presentation of self

2. Given enough time, freedom, and sense of safety, the therapy group evolves into a social microcosm, a miniaturized representation of each member's social universe.
3. A regular interpersonal sequence occurs:

Pathology display: Members display their characteristic maladaptive behavior as tensions and interpersonal interactions in the group emerge.

Feedback and self-observation: Members share observations of each other's behavior, and discover some of their blind spots and interpersonal distortions.

Sharing reactions: Members point out each other's blind spots, and share responses and feelings in reaction to each other's interpersonal behavior.

Result of sharing reactions: Each member begins to have a more objective picture of his or her own behavior and the impact it has on others. Interpersonal distortions become clarified.

One's opinion of self: Each member becomes aware of how his or her own behavior influences the opinions of others and, hence, his or her own self-regard.

Sense of responsibility: As a result of understanding how interpersonal behavior influences one's sense of self-worth, members become more fully aware of responsibility for correcting interpersonal distortions and establishing a healthier interpersonal life.

Realization of one's power to effect change: With the acceptance of responsibility for life's interpersonal dilemmas, each member begins to realize that one can change what one has created.

Degree of affect: The more affectively laden the events in this sequence, the greater is the potential for change. The more that the different steps of interpersonal learning occur as a corrective emotional experience, the more enduring is the experience.

Interpersonal learning is the cardinal mechanism for change in unstructured, longer-term, high-functioning interaction groups. In these settings, in fact, the elements of interpersonal learning are ranked by members as being the most helpful aspect of the group therapy experience (16, 17). Not all therapy groups concentrate in an explicit manner on interpersonal learning; however, interpersonal interaction, with its rich potential for learning and change, occurs any time a group assembles. It behooves the group therapist of every persuasion to be familiar with these fundamental principles.

■ FORCES WHICH MODIFY THE THERAPEUTIC FACTORS

Group therapy is a forum for change whose form, content, and process varies considerably across groups in different settings with different goals, and within the same group at any given time. In other words, different types of groups make use of different clusters of therapeutic factors, and furthermore, as a group evolves, different sets of factors come into play. Three modifying forces influence the therapeutic mechanisms at work in any given group: the type of group, the stage of therapy, and individual differences among patients.

TYPE OF GROUP

Different kinds of groups make use of different therapeutic factors. When researchers ask members of long-term interactional outpatient groups to identify the most important therapeutic factors in their treatment, they consistently select a constellation of three—interpersonal learning, catharsis, and self-understanding (14). Inpatients, in contrast, identify other mechanisms: the instillation of hope, for example, and the existential factor of assumption of responsibility (18, 19).

Why these differences? For one thing, inpatient groups usually have high member turnover and are quite heterogeneous in clinical composition; patients with greatly differing ego-strength, motivation, goals, and psychopathology meet in the same group for varying lengths of time. Furthermore, psychiatric patients usually enter the hospital in a state of despair, after they have exhausted other available resources. The instillation of hope and the assumption of responsibility are most important for patients in this state. Long-term higher-functioning outpatients, however, are more stable and are motivated to work on more subtle and complex issues of interpersonal functioning and self-knowledge.

Groups that are centered around self-help concepts, such as Alcoholics Anonymous and Recovery, Inc., or specialized support groups, such as Compassionate Friends (for bereaved parents), have a clear and focused agenda. In such groups, an entirely different set of therapeutic factors will be most operative, generally those of universality, guidance, altruism, and cohesiveness (20).

STAGE OF THERAPY

Patients' needs and goals change during the course of psychotherapy, and so do the therapeutic factors which are most helpful to them. In its early stages, an outpatient group is concerned with establishing boundaries and maintaining membership, and factors such as instillation of hope, guidance, and universality dominate.

Other factors, such as altruism and group cohesiveness, are salient in outpatient groups throughout the duration of therapy. Their nature, however, and the manner in which they are manifested, changes dramatically with the stage of the group. Consider altruism, for example. Early in the group, patients manifest altruism by offering suggestions to each other, by asking appropriate questions, and by showing concern and attention. Later, they may be able to express a deeper sharing of emotion and a more genuine sharing.

Cohesiveness is another therapeutic factor whose nature and role in the group changes over time. Initially, group cohesiveness is reflected in group support and acceptance. Later, it facilitates self-disclosure. Ultimately, group cohesiveness makes it possible for members to explore various tensions, such as issues of confrontation and conflict, tensions so essential to interpersonal learning. These in turn foster a different, deeper sense of closeness and group cohesiveness. The longer patients participate in a group, the more they value the therapeutic factors of cohesiveness, self-understanding, and interpersonal interaction (17).

INDIVIDUAL DIFFERENCES AMONG PATIENTS

Each patient in group psychotherapy has his or her own needs, personality style, level of functioning, and psychopathology. Each patient finds a different set of therapeutic factors to be beneficial. Higher-functioning patients, for example, value interpersonal learning more than do the lower-functioning patients in the same group. In a study of inpatient groups, both types of patients chose awareness of responsibility and catharsis as helpful elements of group therapy; however, the lower-functioning patients also valued the instillation of hope, whereas higher-functioning patients selected universality, vicarious learning, and interpersonal learning as additional useful experiences (19).

A group experience resembles a therapeutic cafeteria in that many different mechanisms of change are available and each individual patient "chooses" those particular factors best suited to his or her needs and problems. Consider catharsis: The passive, repressed individual benefits from experiencing and expressing strong affect, while someone with impulse dyscontrol profits from self-restraint and an intellectual structuring of the affective experience. Some patients need to develop very basic social skills, while others benefit from the identification and exploration of much subtler interpersonal issues.

■ REFERENCES

1. Fuhriman A, Butler T: Curative factors in group therapy: a review of the recent literature. Small Group Behavior 1983; 14:131-142
2. Corsini R, Rosenberg B: Mechanisms of group psychotherapy: processes and dynamics. Journal of Abnormal and Social Psychology 1955; 51:406-411
3. Yalom ID: The Theory and Practice of Group Psychotherapy. New York, Basic Books, 1970
4. Bloch S, Crouch E: Therapeutic Factors in Group Psychotherapy. Oxford, England, Oxford University Press, 1985
5. Goldstein AP: Therapist–Patient Expectancies in Psychotherapy. New York, Pergamon Press, 1962
6. Bloch S, Bond G, Qualls B, et al: Patients' expectations of therapeutic improvement and their outcomes. Am J Psychiatry 1976; 133:1457-1459
7. Flowers J: The differential outcome effects of simple advice, alternatives and instructions in group psychotherapy. Int J Group Psychother 1979; 29:305-315
8. Bandura A, Blanchard EB, Ritter B: The realtive efficacy of desensitization and modeling approaches for inducing behavioral, affective and attitudinal changes. J Pers Soc Psychol 1969; 13:173-199

9. Yalom ID: Existential Psychotherapy. New York, Basic Books, 1980
10. Budman SH, Soldz S, Demby A, et al: Cohesion, alliance, and out-come in group psychotherapy: an empirical examination. Psychiatry, in press
11. Sullivan HS: Psychiatry: introduction to the study of interpersonal relations. Psychiatry 1938; 1:121-134
12. Goffman E: Encounters: Two Studies in the Sociology of Interaction. Indianapolis, Bobbs-Merril, 1961
13. Alexander F, Franck T: Psychoanalytic Therapy: Principles and Applications. New York, Ronald Press, 1946
14. Yalom ID: The Theory and Practice of Group Psychotherapy, 3rd ed. New York, Basic Books, 1985
15. Yalom ID: Interpersonal learning, in Psychiatry Update: The American Psychiatric Association Annual Review, vol. 5. Edited by Frances AJ, Hales RE. Washington, DC, American Psychiatric Press, Inc., 1986
16. Freedman S, Hurley J: Perceptions of helpfulness and behavior in groups. Group 1980; 4:51-58
17. Butler T, Fuhriman A: Patient perspective on the curative process: a comparison of day treatment and outpatient psychotherapy groups. Small Group Behavior 1980; 11:371-388
18. Yalom ID: Inpatient Group Psychotherapy. New York, Basic Books, 1983
19. Leszcz M, Yalom ID, Norden M: The value of inpatient group psychotherapy and therapeutic process: patients' perceptions. Int J Group Psychother 1985; 35:177-196
20. Lieberman MAL, Borman L: Self-Help Groups for Coping with Crisis. San Francisco, Jossey Bass, 1979

3 BUILDING THE FOUNDATIONS FOR A PSYCHOTHERAPY GROUP

Long before the first meeting of a psychotherapy group, the leader has been hard at work, for the group therapist's first task is to establish a physical entity where none had existed. In this role of founder, the therapist is the group's initial catalyst and its primary unifying force: Members relate to one another at first through their common relationship with the leader and then with the goals and framework he or she has chosen for the group (Table 1).

■ ASSESSING CONSTRAINTS AND CHOOSING GOALS

Every leader would like to establish a therapy group which is stable, meets regularly, and has a homogeneous and motivated membership capable of working toward ambitious therapeutic goals—but in reality, very few clinical situations facing the group therapist meet these ideal criteria. Therefore, therapists must follow two steps prior to formulating goals for a group:

1. They must first assess the intrinsic, immutable clinical conditions or constraints within which the group must work.
2. They must then examine the extrinsic factors bearing upon the group and change those which hinder the group's ability to work effectively.

Once the leader has established the best possible structure for a group, given these intrinsic and extrinsic factors, he or she can then choose appropriate goals.

INTRINSIC CONSTRAINTS

The intrinsic constraints are built into the clinical context of a therapy group; they are facts of life which simply cannot be changed, and the group leader must find ways of adapting to them. For example, patients on legal probation may be obliged to

TABLE 1. **Building the Foundations of a Psychotherapy Group**

1. Assess clinical constraints

   - *Intrinsic clinical constraints:* facts of life, things which cannot be changed, must be incorporated into the structure of group in the most therapeutic manner possible

   - *Extrinsic factors:* things which can be changed by the therapist to make the best possible group structure given the limitations of the intrinsic constraints

2. Establish basic structure for the group

   - Patient population
   - Staff support
   - General time constraints
   - Length of treatment
   - General aim of treatment

3. Formulate specific goals for the group

   - Appropriate to clinical situation
   - Achievable in available time constraints
   - Tailored to capacity of group members

4. Determine exact setting and size of the group

5. Establish exact time framework of the group

   - Frequency of sessions
   - Meeting times
   - Duration of meetings
   - Lifespan of the group
   - Use of open or closed group

6. Decide on use of a cotherapist

7. Combine group therapy with other treatment as indicated

show mandatory attendance at a probation group, and the leader must take this into careful consideration when reflecting upon reasonable expectations for outcome. Motivation levels among probationers in a mandatory group will be very different from those of married couples attending a church workshop on resolving marital conflict. Other intrinsic clinical factors, such as duration of treatment (say, in a medical ward group of hospitalized patients with cancer), also influence the selection of appropriate goals for a group.

EXTRINSIC FACTORS

Extrinsic factors are those which have become tradition or policy in a given clinical setting, and although they appear at first glance to be immutable, they are factors which a therapist can influence as he or she formulates appropriate goals for a therapy group. For example, an inpatient unit may have only one or two group meetings a week which last 30 minutes, but before the therapist chooses limited goals for that unsatisfactory time frame, he or she must first ascertain whether or not these time constraints can be changed so that more ambitious goals can be achieved.

Extrinsic factors are arbitrary and within the power of the therapist to change. Many of them consist of clinical attitudes; for example, the administrative staff of a behavioral medicine clinic may not feel that group psychotherapy is an important part of the clinical program. In such a case, a therapist in the clinic might wish to establish a stress reduction group, but he or she will find it difficult to obtain adequate referrals, space, or clerical support. Therapists must make a vigorous attempt to address and change these extrinsic factors prior to actually establishing a therapy group.

CHOOSING ACHIEVABLE GOALS

After reviewing the intrinsic constraints facing a group, and after modifying extrinsic factors which bear upon the therapeutic work, the leader has a firm grasp of the group's general structure. This includes the patient population, the length of treatment, the frequency and duration of meetings, and staff support (Table 1). The therapist's next step is to shape a set of goals that is appropriate to the clinical situation and achievable in the available time frame. The goals of the long-term outpatient group are ambitious:

to offer symptomatic relief and also to change character structure. An attempt to apply these same goals to an aftercare group of chronic schizophrenic patients will result in therapeutic nihilism. In time-limited, specialized groups, the goals must be specific, achievable, and tailored to the capacity and potential of the group members. Nothing so inevitably ensures the failure of a therapy group as the choice of inappropriate goals.

The group must be a success experience. Patients enter psychotherapy feeling defeated and demoralized, and the last thing they need is another failure because of their inability to accomplish the group task. Furthermore, if leaders formulate unreachable goals for a group, they may grow angry and impatient with their patients' lack of progress, and this will compromise their ability to work therapeutically. The choice of goals for specialized therapy groups is discussed in detail in Chapters 7 and 8.

■ SETTING AND SIZE OF THE GROUP

The setting and size of a therapy group are functions of the relevant clinical constraints. The therapist starting a biweekly group meeting in a halfway house is faced with prospects on group setting and size that are very different from those faced by the consulting psychiatrist arranging a staff retreat for hospital personnel working with AIDS patients.

SETTING OF THE GROUP

It is important for the group therapist to choose a meeting place that is consistently available, of adequate size, with comfortable seating, and that provides privacy and freedom from distraction. This is true for both traditional group psychotherapy meetings and for alternative forms of group work such as staff retreats. The leader must check any meeting places he or she plans to use ahead of time, or the group session can be diverted into a mad scramble to find an adequate room, to locate sufficient chairs, and to cope with unplanned interruptions.

A circular seating arrangement is always necessary: All the group members must be able to see one another. The use of long sofas on many inpatient wards and some casual settings legislates against good interaction. If three or four members sit in a row, they cannot see one another and consequently most remarks get directed to the therapist, the one person visible to all. Obstructing furniture in the center of the room, or having members seated at markedly different levels (some in chairs, some on the floor) obscures direct eye contact and interferes with good interaction.

Some therapists provide coffee and tea at the meeting place, which helps to decrease patients' initial sense of anxiety. This is a useful technique with ongoing groups for lower-functioning patients (such as medication clinic groups for schizophrenics) and for certain short-term groups. For example, in a brief group for bereaved spouses, serving refreshments helped to emphasize the social supportive aspects of the sessions (1).

SIZE OF THE GROUP

The optimal size of a group is linked closely to the therapeutic factors that the leader wishes to foster in the group work. Organizations such as Alcoholics Anonymous and Recovery, Inc., which rely heavily on inspiration, guidance, and suppression to change members' behavior, operate with up to 80 members. In contrast, leaders working in a therapeutic community (for example, a residential halfway house), might make use of an entirely different set of therapeutic factors: They may wish to utilize group pressure and interdependence to foster a sense of individual responsibility to the social community. In this kind of a setting, and with these kinds of therapeutic goals, groups of approximately 15 members are more appropriate.

The ideal size for a prototypic interpersonally oriented interactional group is 7 or 8 members, and certainly no more than 10. Too few members will not provide the necessary critical mass of interpersonal interactions. There will not be enough opportunities for broad consensual validation of different viewpoints, and patients will tend to interact one at a time with the therapist rather than with one another. Anyone who has ever tried to conduct a group with only two or three patients knows the frustration of such an enterprise. In a group with more than 10 members, there may be ample fruitful interaction, but some members will be left out: There will be insufficient time to examine and understand all of the interactions for each of the members.

When working with inpatients, or when leading specialized outpatient groups, the focus will not be as explicitly interpersonally oriented as in the prototypic interaction group—but the therapist must still aim for a lively and engaging group, one that encourages active participation by as many members as possible. The optimal group size that allows members to share experiences with one another ranges from a minimum of 4 or 5 to a maximum of 12; groups of 6 to 8 offer the greatest opportunity for verbal exchange among all patients.

■ TIME FRAMEWORK OF THE GROUP

In group psychotherapy, the leader has sole responsibility for establishing and maintaining all aspects of the time framework of the group within the given constraints of the clinical setting. These include the duration and frequency of sessions, as well as the use of open or closed groups.

THE DURATION OF MEETINGS

The optimal duration for a session in ongoing group therapy is between 60 and 120 minutes (2). Twenty to 30 minutes are required for the group to warm up, and at least 60 minutes are needed to work through the major themes of the session. There is a point of diminishing returns, as after about two hours most therapists find that they begin to fatigue and the group becomes weary and repetitive. This principle also holds true at staff retreats and workshops, where time-limited, more focused sessions are embedded within the context of the overall retreat.

Groups that consist of lower-functioning patients who have a briefer attention span and can only tolerate limited social stimuli, require shorter sessions. Forty-five to 60-minute meetings allow these kinds of groups to maintain their cohesiveness and to focus on a limited number of issues without straining the capacities of more fragile patients. Groups that meet less often or that are centered on higher-functioning interactional work require at least 90 minutes per session in order to be fruitful. Some group leaders allot an additional fixed amount of time for process review or for the observation of therapists' review at the end of each session (2).

FREQUENCY OF MEETINGS

The frequency of group meetings varies widely, again depending on the clinical constraints and therapeutic goals of the group in question. At one extreme are sessions which meet once a day, typically in the inpatient setting, where therapy groups meet optimally from three to six times a week. At the other extreme are once-a-month medication clinic support groups, or once-yearly staff retreats.

A once-weekly schedule is most common in outpatient group work and is well suited to supportive or specialized groups, particularly those that operate with a fixed number of sessions. Ongoing specialized outpatient groups with a limited agenda, such as a narcolepsy support group, generally meet biweekly or monthly. Long-term interactional groups, if they are to be successful, must meet at least once per week; twice-weekly sessions, when feasible, greatly increase the group's intensity and productivity.

THE USE OF OPEN VERSUS CLOSED GROUPS

The decision to run an open or a closed group is closely related to the clinical setting, goals, and identified lifespan of the group. A closed group meets for a predetermined number of sessions, begins with a fixed number of members, and, as of the first session, closes its doors and accepts no new members. Some clinical settings dictate exactly when a closed group must begin and end. For example, in a university health center, a support group for graduate students having trouble with their dissertations must run only for the academic term; class schedules and vacations require that the group begin and end on a specific date. Some closed groups, such as those for eating disorders or for bereavement, have a protocol for a predetermined number of sessions with a specific planned agenda for each session.

In contrast, open groups are more flexible about membership and structure. Some allow for a fluctuation in membership, such as the ongoing inpatient group on a psychiatric ward that reflects ward census, while others maintain a consistent size by replacing members who leave the group. Open groups usually have a broader set of therapeutic goals, and generally meet indefinitely; although members come and go, the group has a life of its own. Even though the members of ongoing outpatient groups may terminate when they achieve their therapeutic goals (on the average, after 6 to 18 months), new members are introduced to take their places. Some groups at psychiatric teaching centers have been known to continue for more than 20 years and to have been the training ground for generations of residents.

■ USING A CO-THERAPIST

Most group therapists prefer to work with a co-therapist. Co-therapists complement and support one another. As they share points of view and examine hunches together, each therapist's observational range and therapeutic power is broadened.

THE MALE–FEMALE CO-THERAPIST TEAM

A male–female co-therapist team has unique advantages. First, it recreates the parental configuration of the primary family which, for many members, increases the affective charge of the group. Second, many patients can benefit from observing a male and female therapist working together with mutual respect and without the derogation, exploitation, or sexualizing that they too often take for granted in male–female associations. More importantly, male and female co-leaders provide the group with a wider array of possible transferential reactions. Patients will differ markedly in their reactions to each of the co-therapists. With a male–female co-therapist team, for example, a somewhat seductive female member may pander to the male leader and ignore his female counterpart, a pattern that would not emerge as clearly in a group led by one therapist. Or a male in the group may ally himself with the female leader in an effort to compete with the male therapist.

Members will have fantasies and misconceptions about the relationship between the male and female co-therapists. These generally relate to thoughts and feelings about the balance of power between the two leaders (who really leads the group?), and to issues of sexuality (do the co-therapists have a sexual relationship outside of the group?). In a high-functioning and cohesive group with skilled and mature co-therapists, these important subjects can and should be explored openly.

CO-THERAPISTS AND DIFFICULT GROUPS

The co-therapy format is particularly helpful for beginning therapists and for experienced therapists working with a difficult patient population. In addition to clarifying transference distortions of each other's presentation in the group, co-therapists support one another in maintaining objectivity in the face of massive group pressure. Often the solo therapist will feel pressured to share the opinion of the group, especially in situations where the therapeutic stance is the unpopular one.

CASE EXAMPLE

Two experienced therapists led a group where a lonely woman member reported that she had become romantically involved with a psychiatric patient on the ward where she worked as a hospital volunteer. She verbally flagellated herself for this in the group session and, in an effort to be supportive, the other members unanimously and vociferously condoned her behavior and attempted to pressure the leaders into a noncritical stance as well. Working together, the co-therapists were able to support one another and maintain their professional objectivity, a stance which ultimately helped the patient to put her behavior into clearer perspective.

Co-therapists are invaluable in helping each other weather an attack from group members. A therapist under the gun may be too threatened either to clarify the attack or to encourage further attack without appearing defensive or condescending. There is nothing more squelching than a leader under fire, saying, "It's really great that you're expressing your real feelings and attacking me. Keep it going!" However, a co-leader can, in such situations, help a patient to channel and express anger at the other leader in an appropriate manner, and then help that member to examine the source and the meaning of that anger.

Co-therapists also help one another to bring up difficult

topics that are remaining hidden in the group, particularly when there is collusion among the other group members to keep these topics covert. For example, in a group where all of the members are deliberately avoiding mentioning an emotional interchange in a previous session, the co-therapists can begin by each presenting their reactions and thoughts about that previous session.

DIFFERENCES OF OPINION

When co-therapists have a difference of opinion during a group session, two factors should be considered: the level of functioning of the group, and the maturity of the group. Patients who are lower-functioning, who are more fragile or unstable overall, should not be exposed to conflict between the co-therapists, no matter how gently it is expressed. Likewise, a beginning interactional group for high-functioning patients is not stable or cohesive enough to tolerate divisiveness in leadership.

Later, in stable, interactionally oriented groups, the co-therapists' honesty about points of disagreement can contribute substantially to the potency and openness of the group. When members observe two leaders, whom they respect, disagreeing openly and subsequently resolving their differences with honesty and tact, they experience the therapists not as infallible authority figures but as humans with imperfections. This aids members who tend to react to others blindly according to stereotyped roles (such as authority figures), and who need to learn to differentiate people according to individual attributes. The group therapy approach is given a powerful endorsement by therapists who are willing to engage personally in the process of open exploration of feelings and resolution of conflict (see the section on therapist transparency).

DISADVANTAGES AND
PROBLEMS OF CO-THERAPY

The major disadvantages of the co-therapy format flow from problems extant in the co-therapy relationship itself. If co-leaders are uncomfortable with each other, or are closed and competitive, or are in wide disagreement about style and strategy, their group will not be able to work effectively. The major cause of failure occurs when co-therapists embrace vastly differing ideological positions (3). Therefore, in choosing a co-leader, it is important to select someone who is different enough in individual style to be complementary, but who is similar in theoretical orientation and with whom there are some comfortable, stable, personal affinities.

Whenever two therapists of vastly different levels of experience co-lead a group, they must both be open-minded and mature, comfortable with one another, and comfortable in their roles as co-workers or as teacher and apprentice. Splitting is a phenomenon that often occurs in groups led by co-therapists, and some patients are very perceptive about tensions in the co-therapists' relationship. For example, if a neophyte therapist feels jealous of a senior co-therapist's clinical experience and wisdom, a member who is intent on splitting might marvel at everything the older therapist says and denigrate the younger therapist's interventions.

Occasionally the entire group becomes split into two factions, with each co-therapist having a team of patients aligned with him or her; this occurs when the patients feel they have a special relationship with one or the other of the therapists, or when they feel that one of the therapists is more intelligent, more senior, more attractive, or has a similar ethnic background or similar problem areas—for example, the recovered alcoholic co-leader of an alcohol recovery group. Splitting, like the problem of subgrouping discussed in a later section, should always be noted and openly interpreted in the group.

■ COMBINING GROUP PSYCHOTHERAPY WITH OTHER TREATMENTS

Group psychotherapy is often combined with other treatment modalities. For example, some of the patients in a group may also be involved in concurrent individual psychotherapy with other therapists; this is conjoint therapy and is the preferable means of combining psychotherapies. In combined therapy, all or some of the members in a group are in concurrent individual psychotherapy with the group therapist. Group psychotherapy can also be combined with brief clinic visits; for example, chronic mentally ill patients at a community mental health center may have a brief session with their caseworker or with the psychiatrist who prescribes their medication, and then participate in a weekly group session.

INDIVIDUAL PSYCHOTHERAPY PLUS GROUP PSYCHOTHERAPY

When is it useful to combine individual psychotherapy with group therapy? Some patients go through a life crisis so severe that they require temporary individual support in addition to group therapy. Others are so chronically disabled by fear or anxiety or aggression as to require individual psychotherapy in order to remain in the group and participate effectively. Individual and group psychotherapy approaches complement each other when the individual and group therapist support one another, are in frequent contact, and when the individual psychotherapy is interpersonally oriented and explores the feelings evoked by current group meetings.

Concurrent individual psychotherapy can hinder group psychotherapy in several ways. When there is a marked difference of approach between the individual therapist and the group therapist, patients may become confused and the two therapies may work at cross-purposes. For example, a patient in dynamically oriented individual psychotherapy, who is being encouraged to free associate and explore childhood memories and fantasies, may become bewildered and resentful when this kind of behavior is actively discouraged in group and when reality-oriented, here-and-now interpersonal engagement is required.

Conversely, the patient who is used to the support and narcissistic gratification of individual psychotherapy, who is accustomed to exploring fantasies, dreams, associations, and memories and to being the exclusive center of attention of a therapist, may become frustrated by the group, especially in initial meetings which often offer less personal support and may be more dedicated to building a cohesive unit and to examining immediate interactions than to deep exploration of each member's life.

Individual psychotherapy and group psychotherapy may also interfere with one another if patients use their individual sessions to drain off affect that would be better expressed in the group. Some patients actively split their two forms of psychotherapy, and compare the support they get from their individual therapist with the challenges and confrontations they experience in the group.

MEDICATION CLINIC SUPPORT GROUPS

Group psychotherapy is used often in medication clinics, a practical and humane combination of treatments generally targeted to those with chronic psychiatric illness. Patients who attend biweekly or monthly medication clinics, usually to receive prescriptions for antipsychotic medication or for lithium, also participate in a group meeting associated with the clinic. Sessions are highly structured and focus on educating patients about their medications and on solving practical problems. Group psychotherapy is used to personalize, enhance, and reinforce the patient's experience in the medication clinic. Research repeatedly has demonstrated the efficacy of group psychotherapy in such aftercare clinics, and in fact there is evidence that the aftercare provided in groups is superior to individually based aftercare (4–6).

■ REFERENCES

1. Yalom ID, Vinogradov S: Bereavement groups: techniques and themes. Int J Group Psychother 1988; 38:419–457
2. Yalom ID: The Theory and Practice of Group Psychotherapy, 3rd ed. New York, Basic Books, 1985
3. Paulson I, Burroughs J, Gelb C: Co-therapy: what is the crux of the relationship? Int J Group Psychother 1976; 26:213-224
4. Claghorn JL, Johnstone EE, Cook TH, et al: Group therapy and maintenance treatment of schizophrenia. Arch Gen Psychiatry 1974; 31:361-365
5. Alden AR, Weddington WW, Jacobson C, et al: Group after-care for chronic schizophenia. J Clin Psychiatry 1979; 40:249-252
6. Linn MW, Caffey EN, Klett CJ, et al: Day treatment and psychotropic drugs in the aftercare of schizophrenic patients. Arch Gen Psychiatry 1979; 36:1055-1066

CREATING A PSYCHOTHERAPY GROUP

After the group therapist has built the foundations for a psychotherapy group, he or she must select and prepare patients who can work toward the goals of the group. The group therapist also has the responsibility of creating a therapeutic environment or culture that permits the new members to work together in a safe and constructive manner.

■ SELECTING PATIENTS AND COMPOSING THE GROUP

Once the therapist has a clear idea of the goals and basic structure of the group—in other words, a clear idea of the group task—he or she must select members who can perform that task. The leader selection and preparation of members is extremely important and greatly influences the entire course of the group.

SELECTING PATIENTS

The therapist's paramount concern in selecting patients is to create a group that coheres. Nothing threatens a group's cohesiveness more than the presence of a grossly deviant member; therefore, the leader selects members who will contribute to group integrity and who will not become deviant in some way. A group of chronic schizophrenic board and care home residents cannot cohere effectively in the presence of a manipulative borderline member any more than a high-functioning group of outpatients can function well together in the presence of a chronic psychotic patient or a patient who frequently goes into dissociative states.

The single most important criterion for selection, no matter what the group, is ability to perform the group task. The study of group failures reveals that deviancy (inability or refusal to engage in the group task) is negatively related to outcome (1, 2). An individual who considers him- or herself, or who is considered by other members, to be "out of the group," a deviant, or a mascot has little likelihood of profiting from the group and has a fair chance of negative outcome.

In clinical practice, the therapist does not actually select patients for a group, but rather de-selects. Group therapists exclude certain patients from consideration (most often because the therapists predict the patient will assume a deviant role or because the patient lacks motivation for change), and accept remaining patients (Table 1). There will be times in a group therapist's career—for example, when running a mandatory inpatient group or a group in a correctional institution—when he or she will have minimal influence over group membership. However, the group leader must always be prepared to exercise the therapist's final prerogative and exclude those patients who are markedly incompatible with the prevailing group norms for acceptable behavior and who threaten the survival of the group. Examples include the physically agitated patient or the manic patient. Patients who cannot tolerate the stress of a group setting, such as the extremely paranoid individual, and patients who are absolutely incompatible with at least one other member, also should not be included in a group. In all of these cases, the therapist has a high degree of certainty that the group will not be useful (and may

TABLE 1. **Selection of Group Psychotherapy Patients**

Inclusion criteria

- Ability to perform the group task
- Motivation to participate in treatment
- Problem areas compatible with goals of the group
- Commitment to attend group sessions and stay for the whole session

Exclusion criteria

- Inability to tolerate group setting
- Tendency to assume deviant role
- Extreme agitation
- Noncompliance with group norms for acceptable behavior
- Severe incompatibility with one or more of the other members

even be harmful) to the deviant patient, and that the therapy of other patients will be jeopardized. Table 1 summarizes basic exclusion and inclusion criteria for group members.

COMPOSING THE GROUP

Suppose that a therapist wishes to start a group for adult children of alcoholics, and is given a waiting list with 15 appropriate referrals. How does he or she decide which patients will work well together? Once again, the therapist must be concerned about the integrity of the physical group. Members must be chosen who are committed to the goals of therapy and are likely to remain in the group.

The key concept to group composition is group cohesiveness. An effective, rough, rule of thumb for longer term outpatient groups is: homogeneity in ego strength, heterogeneity in problem areas (3). A heterodox of personality styles, ages, and problem areas enriches the broth of the ensuing group interaction. For example, in an interactionally oriented outpatient group, members with a range of backgrounds and presenting complaints (say, a young man with issues around success and authority, a middle-aged woman struggling with emotional independence, a young woman seeking to break out of social isolation) will form a group that is rich with many potential avenues for interpersonal exploration. And yet, each member must possess the necessary ego strength to tolerate the affective and cognitive experience of examining here-and-now interactions in the group.

The situation is different in specialized group, when the patients are homogeneous for one major problem area (whether it is an eating disorder, or bereavement, or chronic pain, and so on), although they may be quite heterogeneous in terms of ego strength. Whenever possible, however, the therapist of the homogenous specialty group must aim for similar levels of motivation and psychological-mindedness in the composition of a homogeneous therapy group. It impedes the work of a fast-paced, highly motivated, group of substance abusers to have one or two members who, recovering from a recent cocaine psychosis, are fragile, brittle, and work-avoidant. Likewise, a stolid group of concrete, chronic psychiatric patients can become destabilized if pushed too hard, too quickly by an agitated or a manic individual.

RANGE OF MEMBERSHIP

Group leaders may wish to apply for a wide or balanced range of membership, such as composing a group with an equal number of men and women, or with a wide age range, or with varied interpersonal activity levels. With certain kinds of groups, balancing composition along these basic parameters influences the initial jelling of a group and/or the themes which surface for discussion. The presence of widowers in structured bereavement groups, for example, greatly changed the pace and emphasis of group interactions when compared to group meetings which consisted only of widows (4).

Some groups require a more subtle sort of balancing composition in their membership. A support group for young women business students is, of necessity, going to consist of members sharing the same sex, same general age range, and same career interests. However, the group composition can greatly benefit from a balance of personality styles and activity levels. The presence of one or two gregarious individuals often provides the spark that first ignites a homogeneous group. Aiming for a balanced composition between such members and their more reflective counterparts goes far in maintaining a high level of stimulation in the group.

EXCLUDING INCOMPATIBLE
PATIENTS FROM A GROUP

The leader who is selecting patients and composing a therapy group must learn to spot in advance those candidates who are at risk of becoming deviant members. One reason that this important task is so difficult is that it is not always possible to predict subsequent group behavior from information available in the screening procedure. There is no more valuable information than an account of the candidate's prior experience in groups. The candidate who has had previous failures in group therapy; who is hostile to the idea of group work; who lacks the social skills, psychological mindedness, or attention span to participate in the group task; or who has unrealistic expectations, will probably sabotage the early attempts of the group to cohere (Table 2).

For an interactionally oriented group, the therapist must use

TABLE 2. **Recognizing the Incompatible Patient in Group Psychotherapy**

- Previous failure in group therapy
- Hostile to idea of group work
- Uses group to seek social contacts
- Has unrealistic expectations for outcome of treatment
- Shows manic, agitated, or paranoid behavior
- Unable to participate in group task

---

one or two intake interviews to focus on the candidate's interpersonal functioning: past, present and during the interview itself. The therapist must assess the patient's ability to tolerate various kinds of interpersonal interactions and to reflect upon them. Suitable questions include, "How has the intake interview been for you so far today? Were there any parts that made you uncomfortable? What is it like for you to reveal things about yourself to a relative stranger?" The candidate who is unable to answer these sorts of questions, or who doesn't even understand the meaning of these questions, will quickly be excluded from the interpersonal interactions of the group. Such an individual will impede the work of any group that makes use of interpersonal learning.

■ PREPARING PATIENTS FOR GROUP PSYCHOTHERAPY

One of the group therapist's essential tasks is to prepare patients for the group. Pregroup preparation decreases drop-outs, increases cohesiveness, and accelerates the work of therapy (5, 6). Thorough patient preparation helps to prime members to begin addressing the group task. This, in turn, affects the leader's early work as he or she begins to build a therapeutic culture and to steer the fledgling group toward its goals.

PURPOSE OF PREGROUP PREPARATION

Many patients hold misconceptions about group therapy's worth and efficacy. They feel that it is cheaper or diluted psychotherapy and therefore not as worthwhile as individual therapy. These negative expectations must be addressed openly and corrected in order to engage the patient fully in treatment. Other patients express concerns about procedure and process: the size of the group? the type of members? the amount of negative confrontation? confidentiality?

One of the most pervasive fears is the anticipation of having to reveal oneself and confess shameful transgressions to an audience of hostile strangers. The therapist must alleviate this fear by emphasizing the safe and supportive nature of the group. Another common worry is a fear of mental contagion, of being made sicker through association with other psychiatric patients. Often this is a preoccupation of schizophrenic or borderline patients, though it may also be observed in patients who project their own feelings of self-contempt or hostility onto others.

A cognitive approach to group therapy preparation has several goals:

1. to provide a rational explanation to the patient about group therapy process
2. to describe what types of behavior are expected of patients in the group
3. to establish a contract about attendance
4. to raise expectations about the effects of the group
5. to predict some of the problems, discouragement, and frustration that may be encountered in early meetings (Table 3).

Underlying everything the therapist says is a process of demystification and the establishment of a therapeutic alliance. This comprehensive preparation enables the patient to make an informed decision to enter the therapy group, and enhances commitment to the group even before the first session.

PROCEDURE OF PREGROUP PREPARATION

All group therapy patients, regardless of their clinical situation or level of functioning, must be informed about the time, location, composition, procedure, and goals of the group. In some settings, such as an inpatient ward or a medication clinic group, preparation for group therapy is minimal, and usually is accom-

TABLE 3. **Preparing Patients for Group Psychotherapy**

Purpose of pregroup preparation

- To explain principles of group therapy
- To describe norms for appropriate behavior in the group
- To establish contract about regular attendance
- To raise expectations about helpfulness of group
- To predict early problems and minimize their impact

Procedure of pregroup preparation

- Occurs during first 5–10 minutes of each session in inpatient groups; during 30–45 minutes of intake interview for outpatient groups
- Orients patient to time, location, composition, and goals of the group
- Describes a typical group session in clear, concrete, supportive terms
- Establishes agreement about attendance and about appropriate behavior in the group
- If an ongoing group, provides a description of recent events in the group (e.g., written summaries)
- Notes common early problems (feeling left out, discouraged at lack of rapid change, frustration at not always being able to talk)

plished in 5 or 10 minutes. This does not mean that it is unimportant or can be neglected. Even this very brief preparation will orient patients to the group experience and will provide guidelines about how best to use the group.

For most outpatient groups, preparation is best accomplished over a 30–45 minute period during one or two individual sessions that the leader has with patients prior to beginning the group. These are often intake, or inclusion–exclusion sessions. Once therapists have decided in these one or two sessions that the patient is a suitable candidate for group therapy, they may then proceed to prepare the patient for the group.

Patients have ample primary anxiety and therapists must

avoid adding the secondary anxiety that arises from being thrown into an ambiguous, intrinsically threatening situation. Therefore, the cardinal aim of pregroup preparation is to describe the group in clear, concrete, supportive terms. This provides patients with a cognitive structure that enables them to participate more effectively in the group from the start. If written summaries are used in the group, the therapist may provide new patients with several summaries from recent meetings so that they may become familiar with other members' names and with current themes in the group.

■ BUILDING THE CULTURE OF THE GROUP

Any time a group of people assembles, whether in a professional, a social, or even a family setting, it develops a culture, a set of unwritten rules or norms which determine the acceptable behavioral procedure of the group. In group therapy, the leader must create a group culture in which energetic, honest, and effective interactions take place. A therapy group is unlikely to develop a therapeutic culture on its own, and the leader must devote considerable attention to this task.

HOW ARE NORMS SHAPED?

Norms constructed early in the group have considerable perseverance, and are shaped both by the expectations of the group members as they start the group and by the behavior of the therapist during the early life of the group. The therapist actively influences this process of norm-setting in two different ways: explicitly (by rule prescription and behavioral reinforcement) and implicitly (by model-setting).

Initially, the leader—during preparation of patients for group therapy or in early sessions—explicitly prescribes specific rules for appropriate behavior in the group, such as sharing concerns about body image in an eating disorders group. Once a group gets underway, leaders shape norms more subtly, for example, by rewarding desirable behavior through social reinforcement. If a usually shy member begins to participate, or if members start to offer each other spontaneous and honest feedback, this new behavior is rewarded verbally, or nonverbally through changes in the therapist's body language, eye contact, and facial expression.

The therapist also implicitly shapes therapeutic norms in the group through model-setting. In an acute inpatient therapy group, for example, the leader models nonjudgmental acceptance and appreciation of members' strengths as well as problem areas. In a social skills training group for schizophrenics, the leader might choose to model simple, direct, socially rewarding conversation. No matter what the level and functioning of the group, the effective leader sets a model of interpersonal honesty and spontaneity for his or her group members. But the therapist's honesty always transpires against a background of responsibility: Nothing takes precedence over the goal of being helpful to the patient (see the section on therapist transparency).

GENERAL NORMS OF GROUP PROCEDURE

General norms of group procedure must be actively shaped by the leader at the very inception of the group. The most therapeutic procedural format of a group is one that is unstructured, unrehearsed, and freely flowing. Even in specialized groups that have a specific protocol or agenda, such as a myocardial infarction education group, the therapist must aid members to interact spontaneously and honestly. The leader may need to intervene vigorously to prevent the development of a nontherapeutic procedure, for example, a taking-turns format in which members figuratively line up to present specific problems or life crises one after another. In such an instance, the therapist can interrupt and ask how the procedure of taking turns got started, or what effect it has on the group. The leader could also indicate that the group has many other procedural options from which to choose.

The therapist must also attend to the time boundaries of the group and convey the sense of preciousness of group time (Table 4). Beginning and ending the group on time, having members remain in the room for the entire meeting, warning the group of upcoming absences, and openly discussing members' tardiness or missed sessions, all contribute to group cohesiveness and influence the therapeutic process very early in the life of the group.

TABLE 4. **Maintaining Time Boundaries of the Psychotherapy Group**

The therapist must:

- Ensure that group meetings occur at regular, scheduled intervals
- Begin and close each group meeting on time
- Ask that members arrive punctually and remain in the meeting room for the entire session
- Warn the group of upcoming absences or changes in schedule
- Openly discuss tardiness or missed sessions
- Provide continuity between sessions by calling previous discussions, noting how members have changed over time, observing new and different interactions in the group

THE SELF-MONITORING GROUP

A self-monitoring group learns to assume responsibility for its own functioning, a norm which should be encouraged in every therapy group. Any therapist who has ever worked in a group where the members are completely dependent upon the leader for direction knows first-hand the signs of the passive group. The patients are an audience who have come to see a play, who are waiting for the leader to make the curtain rise and the action begin. The meeting is stilted, heavy, forced. After every session, the leader feels fatigued and irritated by the burden of making it all work.

How can the therapist build a culture which encourages the development of a self-monitoring group? By keeping in mind that, initially, only the leader knows the definition of a productive, hard-working session. Even in a highly structured, specialized group, there is room for patient autonomy and spontaneity. The therapist must start, at the very inception of a group, to share this knowledge with the patients and slowly educate them to recognize a good session: "This was an exciting meeting today and everyone shared a lot. I hate to see it end." The evaluative function can then be shifted to the patients: "How is the group going so far today? What's been the most satisfying part?" And, finally, members can be taught that they have the ability to influence the course of a session: "Things have been slow today. What could we do to make it different?"

SELF-DISCLOSURE

Patients will benefit from group therapy only if they disclose a great deal about themselves. The most useful early guideline to offer patients is that self-disclosure must occur, but at each member's own pace and in a manner that feels safe and supported. The therapist makes these points explicitly during pregroup individual preparation meetings, and actively pursues them during the initial culture-building of the group. For example, during a member's first self-disclosure, the therapist makes frequent and gentle checks to see at what point he or she wishes to stop.

The patient should never be punished for self-disclosure. One of the most destructive events that can occur in a group is for members to use personal, sensitive material, which has been disclosed in the group, against one another in times of conflict. For example, when Bill, a young, aggressive group member, becomes angry at Sue for not siding with him in a disagreement, he may flare up and accuse her of being "basically a disloyal person— after all, you even told us you're involved in an extramarital affair." The therapist must intervene vigorously at this point; not only is this comment hitting below the belt, but it undermines important group norms of cohesiveness, safety, and trust. Any other work in the group must be temporarily suspended so that the incident may be understood and underscored as a violation of trust. In one way or another, the therapist must reinforce the norm that self-disclosure is not only important but safe.

Self-disclosure is always an interpersonal act, and the implications of this, too, must become part of the therapeutic culture of the group. What is important is not that one shares a secret or unburdens oneself, but that one discloses something which is relevant to one's relationship with other members. The therapist must be ready to point out that disclosure results in a deeper, richer, and more complex relationship with others in the group. When a condescending, supercilious patient admits that he has always felt physically and mentally inferior to others, this allows members to understand him better, to feel closer and warmer toward him, and, in turn, the patient can relinquish his pose of superiority in the group.

MEMBERS AS AGENTS OF HELP AND SUPPORT

The group increases in cohesiveness when members come to recognize it as a rich reservoir of interpersonal information and support. The therapist must continuously reinforce the notion that the group functions best when every member is seen as a potential agent of help and support to the others. At times, the leader may have to give up a cherished role as fount of wisdom and expertise or as ultimate arbiter in group issues!

For example, let us assume that a member expresses curiosity about his habit of telling long, rambling anecdotes. Rather than come up with an expert answer, the therapist tells the patient that any information he desires about his behavior is present in the group room, and just needs to be tapped correctly. Or, if a member has been receiving feedback about her domineering and threatening attitude in the group, the leader can go on to ask, "Elizabeth, could you think back over the last 45 minutes? Which comments have been the most helpful to you? Which the least?"

The group functions best if its members appreciate the valuable help they can offer each other. To reinforce this norm, the therapist calls attention to incidents demonstrating the mutual helpfulness or supportiveness of members to each other in times of crisis or need. The therapist also explicitly teaches members more effective ways of assisting one another. For example, after a patient has been working with the group on some issue for a long portion of the meeting, the therapist notes, "I think Anita and Frank offered you some really helpful insights about your depression, Vince. It seems you found their comments most helpful when they were very specific and offered you some alternatives."

CONTINUITY BETWEEN MEETINGS

The ideal therapeutic culture is one in which patients greatly value their therapy group. Continuity between meetings is a means to this end; group sessions take on more weight and value if they are part of an ongoing, evolving process rather than several static punched-out events disconnected from one another. This potent continuity is generally only possible in high-functioning outpatient groups or in certain highly charged specialized support groups (such as a bereavement group). Nonetheless, no matter what the group setting or clinical constraints, the therapist must reinforce whatever continuity exists between meetings in any manner possible.

Therapists can begin emphasizing continuity by sharing thoughts they have had about the group between sessions. Group leaders can also reinforce members when they give testimony of the group's usefulness to them in their ongoing outside life or when they indicate they have been thinking about other members during the week.

A second step is to underline the continuity in group concerns, issues, and interactions as they occur from meeting to meeting. A well-functioning group will continue to work through issues from one meeting to the other, but some groups will need encouragement to reflect upon the themes that weave through the sessions (and that contribute to the building of the social microcosm of each of the group members).

More than anyone else, the therapist is the group time binder, connecting events and fitting experiences into the temporal matrix of the group. "This sounds very much like what John has been working on two weeks ago." Or, "Ellen, I've noticed that ever since you and Judy had that run-in three weeks ago, you've been appearing more depressed and withdrawn. What are your feelings now toward Judy?" If the leader ever begins a group meeting, it should only be in the service of providing continuity between meetings. "The last meeting was very intense! I wonder what types of feelings people took home from the group?" (An exception to this occurs in inpatient groups, where the group leader routinely begins the meeting. See Chapter 7.)

■ REFERENCES

1. Yalom ID: A study of group therapy dropouts. Arch Gen Psychiatry 1966; 14:393-414
2. Connelly JL, Piper WE, DeCarufel FL: Premature termination in group psychotherapy: pretreatment and early treatment predictors. Int J Group Psychother 1986; 36:145-152

3. Whitaker DS, Lieberman MAL: Psychotherapy Through the Group Process. New York, Atherton Press, 1964

4. Yalom ID, Vinogradov S: Bereavement groups: techniques and themes. Int J Group Psychother 1988; 38:419–457

5. Piper W, Debbane E, Bienvenu J, et al: Preparation of patients: a study of group pretraining for group psychotherapy. Int J Group Psychother 1982; 32:309-325

6. Yalom ID: The Theory and Practice of Group Psychotherapy, 3rd ed. New York, Basic Books, 1985

5 RESOLVING COMMON PROBLEMS IN GROUP PSYCHOTHERAPY

Once a group has been formed and has achieved stability, the work of therapy begins. The major therapeutic factors—cohesiveness, altruism, catharsis, interpersonal learning—operate with increasing force and effectiveness, and there is no limit to the ensuing richness and intricacy of group sessions. It is not possible, therefore, to offer specific guidelines through the vast maze of situations and issues that the therapist encounters in a series of group sessions. And yet, certain common concerns occur with sufficient frequency in all groups to warrant specific mention: These include membership problems, subgrouping, conflict, and the handling of problem patients.

■ MEMBERSHIP PROBLEMS

The early developmental sequence and potency of a therapy group is strongly affected by membership problems. Turnover in membership, tardiness, and absence are facts of life in all groups, yet unfortunately these facts threaten a group's stability and integrity. Therapists often find it difficult to confront these issues, perhaps fearing that a firm stance will threaten or definitively chase away the patient who is exhibiting ambivalence toward the group. When therapists turn a blind eye to membership problems, they collude with behavior which diminishes group cohesiveness.

ABSENTEEISM

Absenteeism redirects a fledgling outpatient group's attention and energy from its important early developmental tasks to the problem of maintaining membership. This problem is draining and demoralizing for group members and therapists alike. Members question the value of the group; therapists feel that the survival of the group is threatened, but they are left to address these issues with the patients who are present rather than the offending absent members. Absenteeism also breaks up meeting-to-meeting continuity, and much time is lost in summarizing events for patients who have missed prior sessions.

The therapist often will feel compelled to fix the situation, and in a desperate effort to maintain stable membership, he or she may adopt a posture that is particularly lenient or seductive to the patient exhibiting absentee behavior. This not only reinforces the patient's interpersonal pathology, it also sets the stage for accusations of favoritism from the other group members.

Tardiness and irregular attendance must be discouraged, if not specifically prohibited, in all group settings. When they occur repeatedly early in the life of a group, they should be corrected immediately through simple decree by the leader—regular membership is absolutely crucial for early group survival. Later in the life of a group, tardiness or irregular attendance can be openly interpreted in the light of the group's interactions. Whenever the situation cannot be improved and whenever absenteeism continues to be disruptive, the therapist must remove the offending member from the group.

The situation is radically different in inpatient groups. Here, continual membership turnover powerfully affects the cohesiveness of the setting, but is not due to phenomena which can be interpreted in terms of resistance or interpersonal pathology. With inpatient groups, the therapist must adopt special techniques to minimize the disruptive effects of changing group composition; in part, the problem of absenteeism is circumvented by reframing the life of the group to a single session.

DROP-OUTS

In the normal course of a long-term outpatient therapy group, 10–35% of the members will drop out in the first 12–20 meetings (1, 2). Dropouts are very common in all kinds of groups, and generally consist of those patients who choose to remove themselves after finding they are unable or unwilling to perform the group task. In a group with open membership, the therapist maintains the group census by replacing dropouts with new members.

Dropouts are threatening to the group's stability for several reasons:

1. They drain time and energy as the leaders and members try to keep them from leaving
2. They impede the development of cohesiveness by threatening membership stability
3. They implicitly (and sometimes explicitly) devalue the group

Dropouts are also threatening to the leader, especially to the neophyte, and the therapist may unwittingly become cajoling or seductive in an effort to keep a patient in the group. In time, this attitude becomes antitherapeutic for the group.

When a patient is strongly convinced of his or her desire to quit a group, or when a group has become disrupted by the behavior of a potential dropout despite the therapist's attempts to aid the patient to participate in the group, the leader must help the patient to leave quickly and decisively. The primary responsibility of the therapist is to the group as a whole, and although leaders may choose to refer group dropouts to other forms of treatment, their most important task is to help remaining members feel that the group is a stable, valued source of support and therapy. Therapists accomplish this by gently placing the dropout in context ("Mary found that our bereavement group dredged up too many painful memories for her"), and by providing closure to the event, usually by having the dropout spend part of his or her last session saying goodbye to the group.

The dropout rate is reduced through vigorous pretherapy preparation (3). If the general problems and frustrations that arise early in a group are predicted ahead of time, there is less likelihood that they actually will occur.

REMOVING PATIENTS FROM THE GROUP

The patient whose behavior continually disrupts and impedes the group process is a significant problem for the therapist. Such a patient—who does not work effectively in the group despite the leader's best efforts—will experience one of several negative outcomes (4) (see Table 1).

The therapist must make every effort to change a problem patient's behavior and to permit him or her to become an integrated member of the group. When these efforts fail, the therapist should remove the patient from the group swiftly and mercifully. This is done most effectively in an individual exit interview, in which the therapist attempts to advance alternative methods of viewing the unsuccessful group experience (such as lack of readiness, or poor group fit). This final interview is also helpful for the dropout patient who chooses to leave the group on his or her own.

When a patient is removed from a group by the leader (as opposed to simply dropping out), there is a powerful reaction

TABLE 1. Effects and Outcome for the Disruptive Patient in the Psychotherapy Group

Effects on the group:

- Threatens group cohesiveness
- Demoralizes other members
- Increases anxiety and inhibits participation
- Disrupts normal maturation process of group

Outcome for the disruptive patient:

- Increases patient's sense of interpersonal isolation
- Forces patient into a deviant role
- Decreases motivation to participate in treatment
- Prolongs patient's interpersonal pathology

from the other members. Initial relief is followed by deep levels of anxiety stemming from feelings of abandonment and rejection. The therapist must help members interpret the event in a more realistic and constructive manner: that the best interests of the patient and of the group were not being served, and that the departed patient may benefit more profitably from another form of therapy. The leader assuages group anxiety by continuing to take responsibility for the departing member—through recommending an alternative form of psychotherapy, or by referring the patient to other therapists.

Removing a patient from a group is uncommon and difficult, but it is an extremely important therapeutic step when a disruptive patient clearly is sabotaging the group's work. The necessity of removing a patient from a group is minimized through careful selection (and de-selection) of group therapy candidates.

ADDING NEW MEMBERS

Whenever the group census falls undesirably low in outpatient groups, generally five or less, the therapist should introduce new members. This may occur at any time during the course of the group, but often there are major junctures in the life of the long-term outpatient group when new patients are added. The first of these is during the initial 12 to 20 meetings, to replace early drop-outs. The second occurs after approximately 12 to 18 months, to replace improved, graduating members.

TIMING THE ADDITION OF A NEW MEMBER

The success of introducing new members depends in large part upon proper timing. Group members often do not welcome or assimilate new members easily if the group is in crisis, or is actively engaged in an internecine struggle, or has suddenly entered a new phase of deeper cohesiveness: for example, a group that is, for the first time, dealing with hostile feelings toward a controlling, self-absorbed patient; or a group that has recently developed enough cohesiveness and trust that a member has, for the first time, shared an extremely important secret about childhood incest.

If a group is working well, some therapists postpone the addition of new members even when the census of the group is down to four or five. But in general, it is wiser not to delay the search for new members and instead, to begin promptly screening prospective candidates. A group of only four or five members lacks sufficient critical mass for effective interactions and will ultimately stagnate.

The most auspicious period for adding new patients is when members sense the need for new stimulation. At times, more experienced members will actively encourage the therapist to add new people to the group. The newcomer serves as a new interpersonal stimulus, and can spark new life into a group that has begun to get repetitious.

PREPARING NEW MEMBERS

Patients entering an ongoing group require not only the standard preparation for group therapy, but they also need specific preparation to help them deal with the unique stresses which accompany entry into an established group. New patients entering established groups are daunted by the sophistication, honesty, interpersonal facility, and daring of more experienced members. They may also be frightened or fear contagion, since they are immediately confronted with members who openly reveal more vulnerable or "sicker" sides of themselves than are usually revealed in the first meetings of a new group. The therapist must anticipate for newcomers their feelings of bewilderment and exclusion at entering an unusual culture, and must reassure them that they will be allowed to enter and participate in the group at their own pace.

It is also helpful to describe to the incoming patient the major events of the past few meetings, especially if the group has been going through some particularly intense tumult or discussing especially sensitive issues. If the therapist uses the technique of written summaries, copies of the summaries of the past several meetings should be given to the new member prior to entry in the group.

ENGAGING THE NEW PATIENT

The new patient should be openly and gently engaged in the first meeting or two. In mature groups, one or several of the more experienced members will take this initiative, but at times this task will fall to the group leader. Often it is sufficient merely to inquire about the newcomer's experience of the meeting: "Mark, this has been your first session. What has the meeting felt like for you? Does it seem like it will be difficult to enter the group?"

The therapist should aid the new patient to assume some control over his or her participation. For example: "Shirley, several questions were asked of you earlier. How did that feel? Welcome? Or was it too much pressure?" Or, "Bob, I'm aware that you were silent today. The group was engaged in business left over from previous meetings when you were not present. How did you feel? Relieved? Or would you have welcomed some questions directed at you?"

OTHER THERAPEUTIC CONSIDERATIONS

The number of new patients introduced into a group distinctly influences the pace of absorption. A group of six or seven can absorb a new member with scarcely a telltale ripple. The group continues with only a brief pause in the flow of the work and quickly pulls the new member along into the stream of interactions.

In contrast, a group of four suddenly confronted with three new members becomes overloaded. There is a screeching halt as all ongoing work ceases and the group redirects its energy to the task of incorporating the new members. The therapist who notes frequent use of the words "we" and "they," or hears the labels "old members" and "new members," should heed these signs of schism. Until incorporation is complete, little further therapeutic work can be accomplished.

The introduction of new members can strikingly enhance the therapeutic process of the old members who may respond to a newcomer in highly idiosyncratic styles. An important principle of group therapy is that every major stimulus presented to the group elicits a variety of responses by the group members. Such opportunity is unavailable in individual psychotherapy, but constitutes one of the chief strengths of group therapy.

David, a handsome, arrogant, extremely successful entrepreneur, entered a long-term, high-functioning outpatient group with a stable membership. Within two sessions, he had provoked a flurry of new and stimulating reactions and interactions in what had become a somewhat complacent and compliant, supportive, cautious group. Jim, who had until then enjoyed a powerful leadership role as the young, dominant, and defiant rebel, felt extremely threatened and spontaneously expressed his fantasy of slashing the tires on David's car. Two of the women in the group found themselves romantically attracted to David, while a third, Lucy, found many resemblances between David and her husband, and began relating to him in a confrontational manner.

The different responses evoked in a group setting by a single common stimulus, such as a new member, can only be explained by differences in the inner world, the inner processing of the stimulus, of each member. The investigation of these differences provides a unique window to the inner worlds of each person in the group.

■ SUBGROUPING

A second common problem encountered in group therapy is subgrouping—the splitting off of smaller units. Subgrouping often occurs in outpatient groups, and almost invariably is a part of inpatient groups. A subgroup arises from the belief of two or more members that they can derive more gratification from a relationship with each other than from one with the entire group. This process can hamstring the group work in a subtle but powerful manner, and the therapist must be alert to its occurrence and be ready to confront it when it appears.

THE PROCESS OF SUBGROUPING

A subgroup may exist completely within the confines of the group therapy room, as members who perceive themselves to be similar form coalitions based on age, ethnicity, similar values, comparable education, and the like. Remaining group members, excluded from the clique, generally do not possess effective social skills and do not usually coalesce into a second subgroup. This phenomenon of ingroup versus outgroup is observed most strikingly in inpatient settings.

Subgrouping also can occur outside the group in the form of extragroup socializing. A clique of three or four members will begin to have private conversations, to have coffee or dinner, and to telephone each other and share separate observations and interactions with each other. Occasionally, two members may become sexually involved and keep the nature of their involvement a secret from the rest of the group; ironically, the events of the therapy group often become a special shared topic between the two.

DANGERS OF SUBGROUPING

Complications arise for all members of the group, whether they belong to the subgroup or not. Subgrouping members feel loyalty to their subgroup, keep secrets from the rest of the group, and grow inhibited in their expression of feelings and thoughts. Those excluded from the subgroup may experience powerful feelings of envy, competition and inferiority. It often is exceptionally difficult for members who feel left out to comment on their feelings of exclusion.

In subgrouping based on sexual attraction or courtship, being part of the romantic dyad becomes more important than the group work. A female member who has secretly paired with one of the men in the group may become more interested in appearing attractive to her partner than in having honest interactions with other members; her male counterpart may treat other men in the group as competitors to be vanquished. These members will be disinclined to reveal problem areas that may cause them to appear romantically or sexually undesirable; thus, the group task of honest self-disclosure is sabotaged.

Patients who violate group norms through subgrouping are opting for immediate gratification of needs rather than for involvement in true interpersonal learning and change. Subgrouping that is not examined in the group, whether it occurs within or outside the group session, is a potent form of resistance. It handicaps the therapist and makes a travesty of other members' efforts to be revealing, to give honest feedback, and to participate fully and authentically in the group process.

CONFRONTING SUBGROUPING

The members of a subgroup can be recognized by a striking code of behavior. They agree with one another regardless of the issue and avoid confrontations among their own membership; they exchange knowing glances when a member who is not in the clique speaks; they arrive and depart from the meeting together. In a romantic dyad, flirtatious, seductive, and provocative interactions occur to the exclusion of the rest of the group. Members of a subgroup will also frequently band together and support one another in subtle (and sometimes not so subtle) devaluation of the contributions from other members.

Subgrouping represents a situation that contains both high risk and high gain. It is not the extragroup socializing which is crippling to a group per se, it is the conspiracy of silence around it that becomes dangerous. If the primary task in the group is to examine in depth the interpersonal relationships among all of the members, extragroup socializing inhibits this examination. Important material—the relationship among members who are interacting outside of the group, feelings of exclusion in patients who are not part of this interaction—remains covert, and the task of the group is sabotaged. The therapist must openly identify and confront this process as it occurs in the group.

In pregroup preparation, the therapist attempts to prevent the occurrence of subgrouping by stating that all extragroup behavior must subsequently be brought back into the group for discussion. When it does take place, subgrouping must be explicitly identified and explored: "Leslie, I've noticed that you and Frank are especially supportive of each other, to the point of excluding other members from your interactions." When the powerful issues that give rise to subgrouping are confronted by the group and discussed openly, they can be of great therapeutic import in the very group they were hampering. Confronting subgrouping is of paramount importance for the therapist working with interpersonally based groups, and is far less important in other types of groups.

■ MANAGING CONFLICT IN THE GROUP

Conflict, another common problem in group therapy, is inevitable in the course of a group's development. Like subgrouping, conflict represents a high-risk high-gain process in the group: it can either sabotage or facilitate the group work.

CLARIFICATION OF CONFLICT

Conflict in a group often is signaled initially by the presence of subtle negative interpersonal interactions that range from low-key put-downs, to pointed jokes, condescending remarks, and outright ignoring of a member. Conflict resolution is almost impossible in the presence of this kind of off-target or oblique hostility. As with subgrouping, it is the therapist's task to render overt that which has been covert: "Bob, I've noticed that you've cut off Mary a couple of times today. I wonder if you're not feeling a little angry because of the feedback the women in the group gave you last week."

Only rarely is conflict expressed openly and angrily between group members. When open anger and hostility occur in lower-functioning groups, it usually represents lack of impulse control and/or primitive, chaotic affective expression that is overwhelming to the members experiencing it. This sort of conflict can almost never be harnessed effectively for interpersonal learning.

In mature, high-functioning groups, the ostensible reason for an open attack is often a red herring for the true underlying issues.

CASE EXAMPLE

In an ongoing group for women graduate students in science and engineering, one of the leaders was severely criticized by members for her open and confrontational stance during an earlier meeting, where she had encouraged Kate, a vivacious yet overly controlled woman, to share explicitly some painful feelings evoked by an upcoming family visit. "Since you obviously don't know how we like to do things in here," exclaimed one of the more angry members to the leader, "we'll just have to learn to tell you to shut up!"

This leader was fairly new to the group; she had replaced the therapist who had founded the group, a woman with a very gentle interpersonal style who left in order to pursue other professional activities. Although the group had not once acknowledged a sense of loss or abandonment at the parting of its founding therapist, nor a sense of unfairness or impotence at having to accept someone in her place, the new leader was continually confronted with conflict, disproportionate anger, and criticism in all her early interactions with the group.

USING CONFLICT TO PROMOTE INTERPERSONAL LEARNING

How exactly can conflict be harnessed in the group and used in the service of interpersonal growth? First, the therapist must find the right level for the group at hand. Explosive conflict is threatening and counterproductive for any group of individuals, but too little conflict—especially with higher-functioning patients—leaves the group stagnant, excessively cautious, and superficial. Here, a judicious amount of confrontation, anger, and conflict resolution can provide an affectively charged learning experience for the group members.

Group cohesiveness is the prime prerequisite for the successful management of conflict. Members must have developed a feeling of mutual respect and trust and must value the group sufficiently to be able to tolerate some uncomfortable interactions. The patients need to understand that open communication must be maintained if the group is to survive. All parties must continue to deal directly with one another, no matter how angry they become. Norms must be established that make it clear that group members are there to understand themselves, not to outdo, defeat, or ridicule one another. Furthermore, everyone is to be taken seriously. When a group begins to treat one person as a mascot whose opinions and anger are lightly regarded, the hope of effective treatment for that patient has been all but officially abandoned.

MANAGING CONFLICT AT A THERAPEUTIC LEVEL

Not all groups tolerate the same level of conflict. The open, conflicted confrontation that transpires between two members of a long-term outpatient group would be devastating in a medication group for schizophrenics. Gentle, cautious disagreement may be appropriate in a time-limited group for patients with panic disorder, whereas it could be seen as an avoidance of real feelings in the long-term outpatient group.

Even the same group may not tolerate the same level of conflict at different points in its development. Early, a prototypic group needs to invest its energy in the development of cohesiveness, trust, and support. In its middle phases, such a group begins the constructive exploration of disagreement and confrontation. Much later, as members are terminating therapy, they wish to focus again on the positive, more intimate aspects of the group experience rather than the divisive ones. Therapists should help members to express gentle disagreement early in the life of the group so that anger does not build up to explosive levels later.

Conflict easily gets out of hand, no matter what the group setting. Leaders have to intervene vigorously to keep conflict within constructive bounds. Most often, this includes helping patients to express anger more directly and more fairly and ensuring that everyone gets a turn at responding to the anger. The therapist's goal is to aid every member to learn something from the angry interaction.

CASE EXAMPLE

Sherry, an accomplished professional woman, angrily accused another, more traditionally feminine member, Sue, of taking up too much of the group time. "You make me cringe and turn off completely when you begin your long and involved stories. I think you're just a manipulative wimp who tries to get us all to feel sorry for you." Sue responded by tears and withdrawal. In order to turn this confrontation into a learning experience for the group, the therapist had various lines of questioning to pursue: Why is Sherry so angry, when others are not angry at Sue? Is she envious of Sue (of Sue's marriage? her femininity?)? Why is Sue so passive in her response? Does she feel Sherry is right? Is she afraid that without long stories she would have nothing to say? How do other members respond to this anger? Who is frightened? Who wants them to fight? Who wants them to make peace? For example, why is Butch, one of the male members, bending over backwards to get Sue and Sherry to make up and to say nice things to each other? Is he trying to seduce both of them? Or is he frightened by a woman's anger?

As with any affectively charged experience in the group, the therapist encourages reactions, active feedback, and consensual validation—a consensus of opinion on the true nature and meaning of the conflict—from all the group members.

■ PROBLEM PATIENTS

Each patient's problems are complex and unique, and require many thoughtful, persevering, and careful interventions from the therapist. However, there are some common behavioral constellations, or stereotyped problem patients, which are especially vexing to both the therapist and the group. Although most strategies for coping with problem patients pertain to the outpatient group setting, some of these basic principles can also be applied to inpatient groups.

THE MONOPOLIST

The bete noire of group therapists is the monopolist, a person who is compelled to chatter endlessly about anything and everything, engulfing all the time and attention of the group. The monopolist persists in describing—in obsessive detail—conversations had with others, or complicated incidents from the outside or the past, topics which are only slightly relevant to the group task. Some monopolists hold the floor by assuming the role of junior therapist or interrogator in the group, and still others use enticing sexual material. Extremely histrionic patients often present a series of major life upheavals which always seem to demand immediate, urgent, and lengthy group attention.

REACTION OF THE GROUP

Although a group initially welcomes and encourages the monopolizing patient—who automatically fills in the gaps and provides some activity in the group—the mood rapidly is replaced with frustration and anger. At first, members are disinclined to silence the speaker for fear of not being polite or of not seeming sufficiently sympathetic to the monopolist's story, or because they fear they will incur an obligation to fill the ensuing silence. This quickly turns to irritation as members begin to feel deluged by the one-way monologue.

In addition, the monopolizing patient poses a subtle threat to the fundamental procedural norms of the group. Patients realize they are encouraged to speak up in the group and to be self-disclosing, but here is a patient who speaks a great deal and yet must somehow be silenced. The monopolist is thus a problem which the group, and especially a young group, simply cannot handle on its own.

THERAPEUTIC APPROACHES

As a general rule, the therapist does well to wait for a group to solve its own problems; but in dealing with a monopolist, the therapist must personally and actively intervene: first, to prevent the monopolist from committing social suicide in the group, and second, to address the issue of why a patient who speaks too much must be silenced.

A two-pronged approach is most effective. To start with, the therapist considers the group that has allowed itself to be monopolized. He or she inquires why the group permits one member to carry the burden of the entire meeting. Such an inquiry will startle the group, the members of which have seen themselves up to that point as the passive victims of the monopolist. The leader may wish to note that by their silence, other members have permitted the monopolizing patient to do all the self-disclosing, or to have acted as a lightning rod for the group's anger, thereby absolving the rest of the group from the need to assume responsibility for any of the group's work. Once members openly have begun to discuss the various reasons for their inactivity in the face of the monopolist, they are recommitted to participating in the group task.

Next, the therapist must work directly with the monopolist. The primary message from the therapist to the monopolizer is deceptively simple: "I do not want to hear less from you, I want to hear more." Although each therapist will fashion interventions according to personal style, the essential message to monopolists must be that, through compulsive speech, they hold the group at arm's length and prevent others from relating meaningfully to them—they hide their real self behind a barrage of words.

Generally, the deep-rooted cause of the monopolist's behavior is not well understood until very late into therapy and, in any case, interpretation of the cause offers little help in actual management of the disruptive behavior as it occurs in the group. It is far more effective to concentrate on the patient's manifestation of self and on other members' response to the monopolizing behavior.

THE SILENT PATIENT

The converse of the monopolist, the silent member, is less overtly disruptive but equally challenging for the therapist. Session after session, through stormy group interactions and humorous bantering, the silent patient somehow manages to remain quiet, withdrawn, and uninvolved in the group process.

CAUSES OF SILENCE

Patients may be silent for many reasons. Some experience such shame or such a pervasive dread of self-disclosure that they fear that any utterance will commit them to progressively greater self-revelation. Others feel so conflicted about appearing aggressive, either unconsciously or consciously, that they cannot undertake the self-assertion inherent in speaking in the group.

Some patients, particularly those with certain narcissistic issues, demand nothing short of perfection in themselves and thus never speak in the group for fear of falling short. Others, often members with feelings of contempt for the group, keep their distance or manage to gain a sense of mastery and control by maintaining a lofty and superior silence.

Those patients who are fearful or especially threatened by a specific member in the group may habitually only speak when that member is absent. Some are afraid of displaying what feels to be an overwhelming neediness and remain silent lest they shatter, weep, or appear weak, while still others lapse into a periodic sulk in an effort to punish others or to force the group or the leaders to attend to them.

THERAPEUTIC APPROACHES

Proper management depends in large part on the individual causes of the silence. These can be gleaned in part from the pregroup individual interviews and from the patient's nonverbal cues, as well as from the few verbal contributions he or she may have made in the group. The therapist should attempt to steer a middle ground—allowing each patient to modulate his or her own degree of participation, and yet periodically making an effort to include the silent patient.

One effective means of inclusion is for the therapist to comment on nonverbal behavior; that is, when by gesture, demeanor, or facial expression the patient evinces interest, tension, sadness, boredom, or amusement in reaction to the group's proceedings. Often the therapist may hasten a silent member's participation by encouraging other members to reflect on their perceptions of him or her, and then asking the silent member to validate those perceptions.

Even when repeated prodding, cajoling, and inviting is necessary in order to obtain a silent member's participation, it still is possible to avoid making the patient a passive object by repeated process checks. "Is this a meeting where you want to be prodded? How did it feel when I put you on the spot? What is the ideal question we could ask you today to help you come into the group?"

If, resisting all these efforts, a patient's participation remains very limited even after three months of meetings, the prognosis is poor. Although a silent patient can benefit somewhat from the group by way of vicarious learning, there is a point of diminishing returns. The group will become increasingly frustrated and puzzled as it vainly coaxes, encourages, and challenges the silent, blocked patient. The patient's position in the group will become even more untenable in the face of group discouragement and disapprobation, and he or she will assume a mascot role. Under these kinds of circumstances, the likelihood of spontaneous participation becomes even more remote. Concurrent individual sessions may be useful in helping a patient at this time. If this fails, the therapist should seriously consider withdrawing the patient from the group.

THE SCHIZOID, OBSESSIONAL, OR OVERLY RATIONAL PATIENT

Patients who are emotionally blocked, isolated, and interpersonally distant often seek therapy out of a vague sense that something is missing. They cannot feel, cannot love, cannot play, cannot be angry; cannot cry. They are spectators of themselves: They do not inhabit their own bodies, and they do not truly experience their own experience. These patients are often described as schizoid, sometimes with obsessional traits; they are almost always overly rational in their interactions and responses.

In a therapy group, such a patient has evidence to confirm that the nature and intensity of his emotional experience differ considerably from that of other members. The patient may initially be puzzled at the discrepancy and may conclude that the other members are melodramatic, excessively labile, phony, or simply of a different temperament. Eventually, however, schizoid patients begin to wonder about themselves. They grow to suspect that there is, inside themselves, a vast reservoir of untapped and unexpressed feelings.

REACTION OF THE GROUP

In one way or another, verbally or nonverbally, the schizoid patient conveys this emotional isolation to the other members. Members become keenly aware of the patient's persistent rationality and absence of real emotional engagement. The response of other members proceeds from curiosity and puzzlement through disbelief, solicitude, irritation, and, finally, frustration. They repeatedly ask the patient: "But what do you *feel* about..?" They soon realize that they are, in a sense, speaking a foreign language to the schizoid patient. Eventually, the group begins to tell these kinds of patients what they should feel and what kinds of emotions they should be expressing. Meetings become very predictable as members make their round of attempts to affectively ignite the patient who remains overly rational and distant. Interactions with the patient become increasingly discouraging. Sometimes members mascot the patient as "the refrigerator" or "Dr. Spock," and the patient thus becomes a source of great amusement to the rest of the group—a role which only isolates him or her further.

THERAPEUTIC APPROACHES

There is research evidence that emotional breakthroughs in the group are not effective in changing such patients' behavior (2), and the therapist must avoid joining the rest of the group in this crusade. Instead, there are several graduated activating techniques which, though not dramatic, are in the long run more useful to the schizoid patient.

As a first intervention, the therapist encourages the patient to differentiate among members. Despite all protestations to the contrary, the patient does not feel exactly the same way toward everyone in the group. "John, I noticed that you seemed to listen very intently when Nina spoke today. How did her comments compare with Joan's? Who has been most helpful in the group this meeting? With whom do you feel the most affinity?" The patient can also be asked about differing reactions to each of the two co-therapists.

The leader helps schizoid patients to stay with, and move into, feelings they shrug off as inconsequential or irrational. When such a patient admits, "Well, I may feel slightly irritated," the therapist suggests that he or she remain with those feelings for a moment. "Hold up a magnifying glass to the irritation. Describe exactly what it is like to us. No one ever said you need only discuss big feelings." In addition, the therapist gently cuts off the patient's customary methods of avoidance. "Somehow, you've gotten away from something that seemed important. When you were talking to Julie, I thought you looked near tears. Something was going on inside."

Another extremely useful technique is to encourage the patient to observe his or her own body and somatic sensations. Often the schizoid, obsessional, or overly controlled and rational patient who is not able to experience or describe affect is aware of affective autonomic and somatic equivalents—tightness in the stomach, sweating, cold hands, flushing. Sometimes, noting a change in body position, such as a folding of the arms or a tendency to lean away, can be a helpful indicator of emotional reaction. Gradually, the group helps the patient to translate these bodily feelings into their psychological meaning: "Bill, you fold your arms every time Sally tries to get you to talk. What are those folded arms saying? Give them a voice."

In the group, schizoid patients are both high-risk and high-reward. If they can manage to persevere, to continue in the group and not be discouraged by their inability to change their interpersonal style quickly, they are likely to profit considerably from group therapy.

THE HELP-REJECTING COMPLAINER

The help-rejecting complainer, also known as the "yes—but" patient, has a distinctive behavioral pattern in the group, implicitly or explicitly soliciting help from the group by presenting problems or complaints, and then rejecting or sabotaging any help offered. These patients continually bring environmental or somatic problems into the group, often stories of complex family or work turmoil, health concerns, and the like. In addition, these problems are described in a manner that causes them to appear insurmountable. In fact, help-rejecting complainers take a certain satisfaction and pride from the insurmountability of their problems.

As the group makes heroic and dedicated attempts to come up with various solutions to the patient's plight, the rejection of help becomes unmistakable. This rejection assumes many varied and subtle forms. Sometimes it is an ambivalent "yes—but" response. Sometimes, while the advice is accepted verbally, it is never acted upon; or, if acted upon, the advice inevitably fails to improve the situation of the patient, who reports this back to the group with only slightly hidden satisfaction.

REACTION OF THE GROUP

The effects on the group are obvious. The other members, initially solicitous, quickly become bored and irritated, then frustrated and confused. The help-rejecting complainer appears to be a greedy black hole of complaints, sucking the group's energy and advice. Worse yet, there is no deceleration over time in the patient's demands. Faith in the group process suffers, as members experience a sense of impotence, and further, as they despair of making their own needs appreciated by the group. Cohesiveness is undermined as absenteeism occurs or as patients subgroup in an effort to exclude the complainer.

The behavioral pattern of the help-rejecting complainer is due to highly conflicted feelings about dependency and need gratification. On the one hand, the patient feels helpless, insignificant, and totally dependent on others, especially on the therapist, for a sense of personal worth. Any attention and notice from the therapist temporarily enhances the patient's self-esteem. The opposite—perceived rejection or a feeling of being ignored by the therapist—sends the patient into a downward tailspin. On the other hand, the help-rejecting complainer's dependent position is vastly confounded by a pervasive distrust and enmity toward authority figures, and by envy and rivalry toward other group members.

THERAPEUTIC APPROACHES

A severe help-rejecting complainer is an exceedingly difficult clinical challenge, and many such patients have won a Pyrrhic victory over the therapist and the group by triumphantly failing in therapy. These patients solicit advice not for its potential value but in order to spurn it; therefore, it is a blunder for the therapist to confuse the help asked for with the help required. It is also a mistake for the therapist to express any frustration and resentment, since retaliation completes the vicious circle and lowers the complainer's self-esteem even further.

The therapist must initially mobilize the major therapeutic factors of group therapy in the service of the help-rejecting complainer, encouraging the patient to make use of universality, identification, and catharsis. The role of altruism or of being helpful to others is also a new experience for the help-rejecting complainer.

After membership in the group has taken on value, and help-rejecting complainers care about their interpersonal impact on others, they can be helped to recognize their characteristic pattern of relating and the effect it has on other members. They can be encouraged to try new ways of communicating their needs to the group, new ways of talking to or with the other members rather than at them. Group members can provide feedback on what kind of communication makes them feel closer to the complainer and what kind of communication pushes them away.

Eric Berne considered the help-rejecting complainer pattern to be the most common of all social and psychotherapy group games, and he christened it "Why don't you—yes, but." (5) The use of such descriptive labels, if they are used in a tone of playful and gentle caring, help to make the process more transparent and accessible to group members. Once they can identify the process of "yes—but," members can offer specific interpersonal feedback to the help-rejecting complainer whenever that process occurs.

THE BORDERLINE PATIENT

Group psychotherapists recently have developed an interest in borderline patients for two reasons. First, because borderline patients are difficult to diagnose in a single screening session, many clinicians unintentionally introduce borderline patients into therapy groups consisting of patients functioning at a higher level of ego-integration. Once in the group, the borderline patient poses a severe challenge: The primitive affects and the highly distorted perceptual tendencies of the borderline patient vastly influence the course of the group therapy.

Second, many psychotherapists have concluded that group therapy is the treatment of choice for the borderline patient, particularly if carried out in close conjunction with individual psychotherapy. Furthermore, research evidence indicates that borderline patients highly value group therapy—often more than individual psychotherapy (2).

ADVANTAGES OF TREATING BORDERLINES IN GROUP THERAPY

One of the major advantages of group psychotherapy for the treatment of a borderline patient is the powerful reality testing provided by the ongoing stream of feedback and observations from the other group members. Because of this, the regression of the borderline patient under stress is far less pronounced in group psychotherapy than it is in individual psychotherapy. The patient may distort, act out, or express primitive, chaotic needs and fears, but the continuous and multifarious reminders of reality in the therapy group keep these feelings muted.

The borderline patient's potential for intense and crippling transference distortions or transference psychosis is reduced in the group situation. First, other members correct distorted views of the therapist; at times, the therapist needs to induce this process actively by specifically requesting other members to validate, or, as is more often the case, invalidate, the borderline patient's perceptions.

Second, the transference opportunity is diluted in the group therapy setting. The patient will develop less intense but more varied feelings toward several individuals in the group. Or, if transference feelings become too heated, the borderline patient can temporarily rest, withdraw, or disengage in the group setting in a way that is not possible in a one-to-one therapy format.

In this manner, borderline patients can profit from the therapeutic factor of identification with the leader, without the danger of merging personal boundaries with the therapist or of falling into a transference psychosis. The group provides the patient with an opportunity to obtain greater distance from the therapist, and from that vantage point, the patient is able to observe and internalize aspects of the therapist's behavior. For example, borderline patients may note how the therapist listens and supports members in the group, and they may then go on to incorporate the same behavior into their own relationships with other group members or with other individuals outside the group.

THERAPEUTIC APPROACHES

Individual psychotherapy with borderline patients is marked by a fluctuating and unstable therapeutic alliance. Patients are often unable or unwilling to use individual psychotherapy for personal change, and instead demand primitive gratification or revenge from the therapeutic relationship.

In contrast, the work ethic of psychotherapy is much more readily apparent in a group, and the observation that other members can work in group therapy—that others can pursue concrete goals, manifest changes, and obtain positive feedback for their new behavior—is an important corrective for the borderline patient. The psychotherapist must redirect the borderline patient's attention to this phenomenon over and over again, especially when dealing with a patient who is particularly needy and dependent, and who focuses exclusively on extracting supplies from the people around him.

Although there is a potential for borderline patients to feel wounded in group meetings when confronted by other members, the ultimate message is that other group members take them seriously and respect their ability to assume responsibility for their actions and to change their behavior. The therapist must continually encourage the group to take this stance toward the borderline patient. If the group responds only to the borderline patient's facile tendency to feel wounded or rejected, or if the group begins to fear the borderline patient's primitive anger, group psychotherapy fails. The group will no longer provide honest feedback to the patient, and he or she will assume a noxious, deviant role.

The borderline patient's core problems lie in the sphere of intimacy and self-integration, and the therapeutic factor of cohesiveness is of decisive importance. If the patient is able to accept the feedback offered by the group and if his or her behavior is not so disruptive as to create a deviant or scapegoat role, then the group becomes an enormously supportive refuge. This resource is especially important for fragile borderline patients who are easily overwhelmed by the stresses of everyday life.

Once such patients develop trust in the group, they may serve, surprisingly, as major stabilizing influences. One will often hear borderline patients proudly refer to the therapy group as "my group." Because it represents the only stable, supportive aspect of their environment, and because borderline patients suffer from severe separation anxiety, these patients often work hard to keep the group together, serving as the most faithful attendees and chiding other members for being late or absent.

The patient's sense of belonging is augmented by the fact that a borderline patient, when not unduly disruptive, is often a great asset to the therapy group. Group leaders frequently note that the patient's easy access to unconscious needs, fantasies, and fears can loosen up a group that is overly controlled. The borderline patient's associations to the group process provide invaluable material and facilitate the therapeutic work, especially in the face of fellow members who are more inhibited, constricted, or repressed.

FINAL CAVEATS

The borderline patient's tendency to distort interpersonal interactions and this patient's general vulnerability to real or perceived rejection are so great that additional conjoint or combined individual psychotherapy is nearly always required. This use of combined psychotherapies is most successful when the group leader and the individual therapist are in close communication, and when the individual therapy is oriented toward interpersonal understanding. The most common reason for treatment failure with borderline patients in psychotherapy groups is the omission of adjunctive individual psychotherapy (6).

Despite recent efforts toward diagnostic precision, the term "borderline" often conveys little information about the salient behavior of the flesh-and-blood individual. Thus, the decision as to whether to include a borderline patient in a group depends more upon the personality and characteristics of the particular person being screened than upon the broad diagnostic category per se. The therapist must assess not only a patient's ability to tolerate the interactional intensity of the psychotherapy group, but also the group's ability to tolerate the interpersonal demands and regressive tendencies of that particular patient.

The work with the borderline patient generally consumes significant time and energy, and most heterogeneous groups can tolerate, at best, only one or two borderline patients. Patients who are grandiose, contemptuous, highly antagonistic, or extremely narcissistic do not have a bright future in the group, and the patient must have the capacity to tolerate minimal amounts of frustration or criticism without indulging in emotional blackmail or serious acting out. With these caveats in mind, however, the borderline patient may often be treated successfully in group psychotherapy.

THE ACUTELY PSYCHOTIC PATIENT

The therapy group is severely challenged when a member becomes acutely psychotic in the course of treatment. The fate of the acutely psychotic patient, the response of the other members, and the effective options available to the therapist all depend upon when the psychosis occurs in the history of the group and upon what role the patient has held in the group. In an older, more established, and mature group—especially one in which the patient has occupied a valued role—the group members are more likely to be supportive and effective in the crisis.

INVOLVING THE GROUP

When faced with a patient who has become acutely psychotic in a group, many psychiatrists reflexively revert to their medical model and symbolically dismiss the group by intervening forcefully in a one-to-one fashion. In effect, they say to the group, "This is too serious for you to handle." Such a maneuver can, at times, be antitherapeutic: The patient is frightened even further by the change in attitude and role of the therapist, and the group as a therapeutic force is diminished.

A mature and cohesive group is perfectly able to deal with the psychiatric emergency of an acutely decompensating member. Although there may be several false starts, the group will eventually consider every contingency and take every action the therapist would have considered. At times, the group chooses the appropriate intervention, such as reassuring the acutely psychotic patient and aiding him or her to seek hospitalization. At other times, the group agrees that the therapist must assume a leadership role and act decisively.

Members of a psychotherapy group who actually participate in planning a course of action are more committed to the enactment and follow-up of that plan. They will, for example, commit themselves more fully to the overall care of an acutely psychotic member and, more importantly, to his or her later re-entry into the group if they recognize that the care of the patient is also their problem and not the therapist's alone.

THERAPEUTIC CONSIDERATIONS

The experience of witnessing a member develop an acute psychosis creates personal upheaval in some, if not all, members. Feelings of guilt at perhaps having provoked the psychosis intertwine with the fear that they, too, can lose control and slide into a similar abyss. Members will feel angry at the acutely psychotic patient for disrupting the flow of the group process and changing the regular format and expectations for the group session. They will express concern over the patient's apparent fragility, and they will wonder about the patient's prognosis for re-entry into the group.

There may be some unexpected benefits for a group when one of its members experiences a psychotic decompensation; group cohesiveness is strengthened when members share intense emotional experiences and master them successfully. However, in general, the group pays a heavy toll for the experience, especially if the psychotic patient consumes a massive amount of energy for a prolonged period of time (in practical terms, this means for more than one session). Other members may drop out, and the group may deal with the disturbed patient in a cautious, concealed manner or simply attempt to ignore the psychotic symptoms, all of which aggravate the problem.

One of the worst calamities that can befall a psychotherapy group is the presence of a manic or hypomanic member. Hypomanic or manic patients overwhelm the other members with their grandiosity, irritability, and unfocused energy; they consume the bulk of the group's time and energy without deriving any benefit from it. They also frequently indulge in very chaotic or manipulative interpersonal interactions ("I don't understand why the leaders in here are telling me to not talk as much or to go easier in my comments—you guys are here to help me and I should feel comfortable telling you everything I feel, right?").

In such critical situations, the therapist must intervene rapidly, instituting appropriate pharmacotherapy, if indicated. The leader may need to see the disturbed patient in individual sessions for the duration of the crisis. Here, too, the group should explore the implications thoroughly and share in the decision, unless the member is so disruptive that he or she must be withdrawn from the group as swiftly as possible.

■ REFERENCES

1. Yalom ID: A study of group therapy dropouts. Arch Gen Psychiatry 1966; 14:393-414
2. Yalom ID: The Theory and Practice of Group Psychotherapy, 3rd ed. New York, Basic Books, 1985
3. Connelly JL, Piper WE, DeCarufel FL, et al: Premature termination in group psychotherapy: pretreatment and early treatment predictors. Int J Group Psychother 1986; 36:145-152
4. Dies RR, Teleska PA: Negative outcome in group psychotherapy, in Negative Outcome in Psychotherapy. Edited by Mays DT, Franks CM. New York, Springer Publishing Company, 1985
5. Berne E: Games People Play. New York, Grove Press, 1964
6. Horwitz L: Group psychotherapy for borderline and narcissistic patients. Bull Menninger Clin 1980; 44:181-200

TECHNIQUES OF THE GROUP PSYCHOTHERAPIST

6

Though individual and group psychotherapists often use similar psychotherapeutic techniques—such as empathic listening, nonjudgmental acceptance, and interpretation—there are a number of interventions that are specific to group psychotherapy. These include working in the here-and-now, using therapist transparency, and employing various procedural aids that enhance the group work.

■ WORKING IN THE HERE-AND-NOW

All groups, even those without direct leadership (for example, a self-help group with no designated leader), can develop an environment where most of the therapeutic factors, from universality to altruism, are operative. The therapeutic factor of interpersonal learning, however, occurs only in those groups led by a trained psychotherapist.

Interpersonal learning in group psychotherapy requires a leader who is well versed in the specific therapeutic techniques of working in the here-and-now. In general, the principles of working in the here-and-now and the use of interpersonal learning are of greatest consequence in prototypic interactional groups, but these concepts can be modified to suit the needs of other kinds of groups and form an essential part of any group therapist's armamentarium (1–3).

IMPORTANCE OF THE HERE-AND-NOW

The primary goal of the long-term outpatient therapy group and, to a lesser extent, of many other kinds of groups, is to help each individual understand as much as possible about his or her interactions with the other members of the group, therapists included. To accomplish this, the members must learn to focus upon the immediate interpersonal transactions occurring in the group.

FOCUSING ON THE PRESENT

The most fundamental principle of technique for the group psychotherapist is to focus on the present, on what transpires in the room in the here-and-now of the group session. By directly focusing on the here-and-now, the leader engages the active participation of all of the members, and in so doing maximizes the power and efficiency of the group. The therapist emphasizes to the group that the most important transactions are the ones occurring in the group room, under the eyes of each and every member.

The therapy group focus is most powerful if it is unhistoric, if it de-emphasizes the historical past and even the current outside life of the individual members, in favor of the here-and-now in the group. De-emphasis does not imply that history is unimportant, only that groups work most efficiently on the interactions occurring in the immediate present, where each member has an opportunity to experience and examine those interactions.

AFFECT-EVOCATION AND AFFECT-EXAMINATION

A group experience must, if it is to be therapeutically effective, contain both an affective and a cognitive component. The group members must be involved with one another in an affective matrix: They must interact freely, they must reveal a great deal of themselves, and they must experience and express important emotions. But they must also step outside of that experience and examine, understand, and integrate the meaning of the emotional experience they have just undergone. Thus, a here-and-now focus consists of a rotating sequence of affect-evocation followed by affect-examination (4, 5).

The absence of either the affective or the cognitive components of the here-and-now experience jeopardizes therapy. Encounter groups often were powerful and exciting events in the 1960s and 1970s, but participants found that a strong emotional occurrence without subsequent examination promoted little real learning. No real therapeutic change occurs unless group members can integrate what they have learned in the here-and-now and then transfer that learning to their real-life situation. Likewise, leaders who focus exclusively on explanations and intellectual integration end up squelching all expression of spontaneous affect and create a lifeless, sterile group.

These are the two stages of the here-and-now focus: affect-evocation followed by affect-examination (Figure 1). Each is important, but they are different in character and demand two very distinct sets of techniques:

1. For the first stage, the stage of emotional experience, the therapist needs a set of techniques that plunge the group into its immediate interactions.
2. For the second stage, clarification of the emotional experience, the therapist needs a set of techniques that helps the group transcend itself to examine and interpret its own experience.

PLUNGING THE GROUP INTO THE HERE-AND-NOW

In order to plunge the group members into active, vigorous, and honest transactions with one another, the therapist must first educate members about the nature and importance of these transactions during pregroup preparation, and later, must focus the group continuously on the immediate present.

TEACHING MEMBERS ABOUT THE HERE-AND-NOW APPROACH

The starting place for shaping a here-and-now focused group is in the pregroup preparation. By using straightforward instruc-

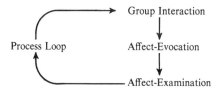

FIGURE 1. **The Here-and-Now Technique of Group Psychotherapy**

tion, the leader offers the patient a rationale for the here-and-now approach through a brief, simplified discussion of the interpersonal approach to therapy. Patients benefit from an explicit description of how various kinds of psychological problems arise from (and are manifested in) their relationships with others, and how group therapy is an ideal setting to take a close look at interpersonal relationships.

Without this kind of explicit preparation, patients become confused by the here-and-now focus of the group. After all, they sought therapy to deal with dysphoric feelings such as anxiety, anger, or depression. How can they not be puzzled to find themselves in a group where the therapist is asking them to reveal their feelings toward seven strangers? To alleviate this kind of confusion and to insure that patients participate fully, some sort of cognitive bridge must be provided for members. This kind of teaching also allows patients to see that the therapist has a rational, coherent approach to the group therapy endeavor.

REINFORCING THE HERE-AND-NOW FOCUS

After laying these foundations for the here-and-now focus in the initial pregroup preparation, the leader continues to reinforce this focus throughout therapy. Experienced group therapists think "here-and-now" at all times, and consider themselves as shepherds keeping the group at work grazing on current interactions. All strays into the past, into outside life, or into intellectualization, must be gently herded back into the present. Whenever the group engages in some there-and-then discussion ("My first husband used to get real abusive to me when he drank"), the group leader must find ways to bring members back into the here-and-now: "Ellie, what brings that to mind for you in the group today? Have you been feeling that some of the men in here are not treating you as gently as you'd like?"

The first session

The therapist begins to steer the group into the here-and-now in its very first session. Consider for a moment the beginning of any therapy group. Typically, some member gets things started by sharing with the group a major life problem or concern and the reasons why he or she is now in this therapy group. Usually this disclosure begets both support and some similar disclosure from others, and in a short period of time the group members have begun to share a great deal.

To plunge the group into the here-and-now, the interaction-ally oriented therapist intervenes later in the meeting with a comment such as: "This group has made a good start today. Many of you have shared some important things about your-selves. But I wonder if something else has been happening here. (And of course the therapist knows perfectly well that something else has been happening.) Each of you has found yourself in a roomful of strangers. No doubt you've been watching each other and sizing up one another and having first impressions." By this time, people in the group are paying close attention, and the therapist then sets the task of the group: "Perhaps we could spend the rest of the meeting today in discussing what your first impres-sions are." Or in a more fragile, lower-functioning group where members would find this open-ended task threatening, an alterna-tive suggestion could be: "Perhaps we could share what we liked the most about each other's participation so far."

These are not subtle interventions. They are heavy-handed, explicit instructions to begin the process of here-and-now interac-tion. And yet the vast majority of groups, no matter what their composition or orientation, respond favorably to this intervention. Even groups of hospitalized patients, if proper boundaries are placed, accomplish this task with considerable ease and benefit.

Encouraging here-and-now self-disclosure

Group psychotherapists must be active and diligent if they are to keep the group discussion in the here-and-now. They must shift the content of the material from outside the group to inside the group, from abstract reflections on problems to specific rev-elations, from generic statements to personal disclosure. If a pa-tient reports that he is too frightened to attend parties because he always says stupid things, the therapist can ask what "stupid" things he has said today in the group. When a patient states that she is embarrassed to talk about certain things in the group, the therapist might ask what the patient anticipates happening if she were to take the risk and talk about something "embarrassing." If a patient who is worried about self-disclosure supposes that peo-ple might laugh or be judgmental, the leader then asks, "Who here in the group would laugh at you?" Once the group member reveals his or her guesses about others' reactions, the door is open to good interactional work. Other group members can confirm or, as is far more often the case, dispute, those guesses.

Identifying an in-group analogue for out-group problems

A basic principle in activating the here-and-now is to identify an in-group analogue for some out-group problem and then to work on the in-group analogue rather than the out-group situation. If, for example, a male patient brings in an account of a fight he had with his wife in which she accused him of being unfeeling, the group leader must search for some type of here-and-now manifestation of that conflict. The therapist might turn the group's attention to some recent meetings, when members complained that this patient was not really empathetic to their problems. Or the therapist might ask some of the female members to picture being married to this patient; to what degree could they imagine being in close emotional contact with him? Without an intervention of this sort, the group will spend its energies on helping the patient solve the reasons for the fight with his wife—an extremely ineffective way to use a group. Generally, when presented with incomplete or biased data, groups are almost always destined to fail to solve outside problems, and members end up feeling frustrated or discouraged.

Interactional implications of ingroup behavior

The therapist who is experienced in working in the here-and-now is able to use almost every incident in the group as a springboard into interactional exploration. If a patient monopolizes the group with a 20-minute convoluted account of a childhood event, the leader should attempt to understand the interactional aspects of this behavior. The leader may remind the patient that he said, in the first session, that he often feels others don't listen to him. "Is it possible," the therapist could ask, "that this is one of those times?" Another tack might be to raise the question of why the patient chooses to deliver this monologue today in the group. "What do the other group members think? Could it be related to a feeling of being misunderstood in last week's meeting?" Or the patient could be encouraged to stop the monologue and to venture a guess as to how the other members are reacting to what he is saying at this moment. Any of these approaches have the same effect: they move the group members away from a content-oriented monologue in which they cannot participate to a discussion of the relationships among members.

Making the here-and-now safe and rewarding

Individuals do not engage naturally and easily in the here-and-now. It is new and frightening, especially for the many patients who have not previously had close and honest relationships, or who have spent their lives keeping certain thoughts and feelings—anger, pain, intimacy—covert. The therapist must offer much support, reinforcement, and explicit training. A first step is to help patients understand that the here-and-now focus is not synonymous with confrontation and conflict. In fact, many patients have problems not with anger or rage, but with closeness and the honest and nondemanding or nonmanipulative expression of positive sentiments. Accordingly, it is important early in the group to encourage the expression of positive feelings as well as critical ones.

The leader must teach group members how to request and how to offer useful feedback that is relevant to the group's interactions, that is specific, and that is personal. Observations or requests that have to do with there-and-then problems or that are global and abstract—such as "What should I do about my fights with my boyfriend?" or "You're a really nice person" or "Am I an interesting woman?"—are always unhelpful. The more specific the question or feedback, the more useful and potent it is. Much more useful are requests such as, "I'd like to explore why I keep locking horns with the men in this group" and feedback such as, "I am most interested and feel closest to you when you share your pain with me, but I get turned off when you present yourself as having it all together and needing very little from the group."

UNDERSTANDING THE HERE-AND-NOW

The second stage of the here-and-now focus requires an entirely different set of functions and techniques on the part of the therapist. If the first stage demands activation and plunging the group into its immediate affective experience, the second stage demands reflection, explanation, and interpretation. This phase of the group work is referred to as group process. If several individuals engage in a discussion, the content of their discussion is obvious: it consists of the actual words spoken and the substantive issues addressed. But the process of the discussion is entirely different. The process refers to how this content is expressed and what it reveals about the nature of the relationship among the individuals who are holding the discussion.

ATTENDING TO GROUP PROCESS

The group therapist must always attend to the process of the communication in a group—must listen to the group discussion with an ear that is examining how the words exchanged shed light upon the relationships among the participants. Consider, for example, the patient who suddenly reveals to the group that, as a child, she was sexually molested by her stepfather. The group members will probably probe for more "vertical" disclosure: They will ask for details about the molestation, for how long the abuse lasted, what role her mother played, and whether it affected her relationship with men.

A process oriented psychotherapist is more concerned about "horizontal" disclosure (that is, disclosure about the disclosure) and, accordingly, will attend to the relational, here-and-now aspects of her disclosure. The leader will consider such issues as: Why is Betty revealing this to us today rather than some other day? What has permitted her to take this risk today? What prevented her from telling us this earlier? How does she anticipate the group will respond? Whose reaction was she particularly concerned about?

The recognition of process is part of the art of psychotherapy and requires a long apprenticeship. To understand process, one needs to register continually all the available data: Who chooses which seats? Who is always late? At whom do members look when talking to each other? Who meets with whom at the end of the group? How does the group change when a particular member is absent?

Some of the most valuable data are the therapist's own reactions and should be put to work. If the therapist feels impotent or frustrated or bored in a group session, it is very likely that many other group members feel the same way. Likewise, when the leader feels engaged or excited by the group interactions, this is often the sign of a potent, hard-working meeting.

RECOGNIZING BASIC GROUP TENSIONS

In order to recognize and understand the process in the here-and-now, the therapist should keep in mind that certain tensions are present to some degree in every therapy group. One of the most fundamental of these is the struggle for dominance. Others include basic group conflicts faced by each member:

1. the conflict between sibling rivalry and the need for mutual support
2. the conflict between greed and the desire to help another person
3. the conflict between the wish to immerse oneself in the comforting body of the group and the fear of losing one's precious autonomy

The therapist who is able to recognize and demonstrate these basic tensions when they manifest themselves in the group can keep the group working effectively. As a clinical example, an articulate and provocative young man long enjoyed the role of the dominant member of a group. When an older, very successful, and aggressive man joined as a new member, the younger man gradually became withdrawn, depressed, and, soon after, announced his intention of quitting the group. It was not until the therapist called attention to the struggle for dominance that the patient began to explore some of his feelings of competition and envy toward the new member.

MASS GROUP PROCESSES

At times there arise situations in which the entire group is dominated by an emotion that is contagious, that vastly influences the work of the group, even to the point of submerging individual dynamics. Two such cases have already been described: the presence of an acutely psychotic member, a situation which may move the entire group into a helpless, dependent position; and the removal of a deviant member, which may result in a resistant or anxious group.

Wilfred Bion developed a model which some group therapists have found useful in understanding mass group processes.
Bion described three basic, recurring, mass-group emotional
states (6):

1. *Pairing* occurs when a group is in an optimistic or a hopeful,
   anticipatory state. Group members often pair up supportively,
   and act as if their aim is to preserve the group by finding
   strength or a new leader from their peer membership.
2. *Dependency* occurs when a group is in a helpless or an awed
   state. Members act as if their aim is to obtain support, nurtur-
   ance and strength from someone outside their peer membership, generally the designated leader.
3. *Fight–flight* takes place when a group is in an aggressive,
   hostile, or fearful state. Here, members act as if their aim is
   to avoid something in the group by either entering into conflict
   or avoiding the task at hand.

The stages of development of a group influence the mass
group states or processes encountered at any given time. For
example, a newly formed, high functioning outpatient group did
well through its first 16 sessions and entered into a productive but
threatening exploration of conflict and confrontation among
members. When a new patient, a vaguely threatening, competitive, and seductive young woman was introduced into the group,
members suddenly consolidated and forgot all their differences
and conflicts. This is in contrast to earlier sessions, in which the
group had absorbed two new members with scarcely a ripple and
immediately drawn them into the comfortable early task of establishing cohesiveness.

Two types of mass group processes arise as obstacles to the
progress of the entire group:

1. those which involve anxiety-laden topics
2. those which involve antitherapeutic group norms

In the first, a topic arises that is so threatening to the group on
either a conscious or an unconscious level, that the group refuses
to confront the problem openly and instead takes evasive action,
referred to as group flight:

Case Example

In a dynamic, cohesive support group for women students attending business school, there was a sudden change in leadership when one of the co-therapists, a psychiatry resident, was rotated off-service without giving the group adequate notice. Two meetings later, members spent an entire session talking about serious illnesses in their families, recent deaths of grandparents, and past losses of close family and friends—there was a great deal of spontaneous emotion, and two usually reserved members wept when recalling the death of a cherished grandparent. There was no mention of the change in group leadership, and when the new co-therapists attempted to bring up the topic, members devoted themselves even more vigorously to recounting stories from their outside lives.

The other mass group process that blocks the group work is the development of antitherapeutic group norms. At one extreme, this includes the development of severe counterdependency—a group which resists all of the therapist's suggestions or interpretations. As in the clinical vignette above, the process of resisting interpretations is often intertwined with the desire of the group to avoid confronting anxiety-laden topics. In an angry, activated group of medical students, for example, members vehemently rejected en masse the leader's suggestions that part of their anger stemmed from personal fears about death, impotence, and decay: "We're not upset about any of that stuff; we're disgusted at how the residents we're working with act so arrogantly toward their indigent patients."

Groups may also develop the opposite, but equally antitherapeutic norm of extreme dependency, a situation in which the leaders are seen as magical, potentially dangerous figures, and the group consistently imbues them with unrealistic power and refuses to approach them as real human beings. Or a group may develop rules which legislate against the recognition or development of intermember tension. In a support group for single parents, for example, the culture of the group was one of extreme sensitivity and deference; the group as a whole not only suppressed any differences of opinion or conflict that emerged between members, it refused to permit members to acknowledge and identify their personal tastes and preferences.

The therapist must decide when to emphasize the interpersonal aspects of an interaction and when to emphasize the mass group process. As a rule, any time an issue arises that is critical to the existence or therapeutic functioning of the entire group, a mass group intervention must be made. The therapist describes the process that he or she is observing to the group using one of two approaches:

1. by identifying and labeling the group resistance specifically— i.e., by making a specific comment about the existence or nature of a mass group process that is preventing the group from dealing with the real issue at hand (for example, by commenting on the way in which sadness over a grandparent's death may symbolize sadness for the loss of a therapist in the group for women business students); or,
2. by pointing out the effects of the resistance—i.e., by observing that the current mass group process might be having deleterious effects on the various members or on the group at large ("I think Anna and Lynne need to explore what seems to be a very real difference of opinion, but people keep changing the subject. Somehow we have developed a group where it's impossible for us to talk constructively about our differences.")

Mass group interpretations are but one small aspect of the therapeutic role of the group leader. In fact, some research has shown that therapists who limit their observations only to mass group comments are ineffectual. Interventions made to the group as a whole are far less likely to instigate self-examination or interpersonal interaction than are interventions made to an individual member or to a dyad (7, 8).

■ USING TRANSFERENCE AND TRANSPARENCY

The transference that different group members develop toward the leader is a powerful event with great therapeutic potential: A member's stereotyped or unrealistic reaction to the leader can be examined and appraised by all of the other group members. In addition, the therapist can use transparency—his or her own reactions, openness, and honesty—to respond to members and to clarify unrealistic expectations and reactions in the group.

TRANSFERENCE IN THE PSYCHOTHERAPY GROUP

A realistic source of strong feelings toward the group leader lies in the members' explicit or intuitive appreciation of the great power that group therapists wield. The therapists' consistent presence and impartiality are essential for group survival and stability. They cannot be deposed. They can add new members, expel old members, and mobilize enormous group pressure around any issues they wish.

However, group members regard group therapists in an unrealistic light as well. True transference or displacement of affect from a prior object, say early parental figures, is one source. Conflicted attitudes toward authority—for example, dependency, autonomy, rebellion—which become personified in the leader, are another. And still another source is the patient's tendency to imbue psychotherapists with superhuman features, such as ultimate wisdom about human nature, so as to use them as shields against existential anxiety.

AVOIDING UNDUE EMPHASIS ON TRANSFERENCE

True transference as understood in psychodynamic terms does occur in psychotherapy groups. Indeed, it is powerful and radically influences the nature of the group interactions. But just as in any group there will be patients whose therapy hinges on the resolution of transference distortion, so there will also be many others whose improvement depends upon interpersonal learning stemming not from transferential work with the therapist but from peer-oriented work with another member around such issues as competition, exploitation, or sexual and intimacy conflicts.

Some therapists, particularly those with traditional psychoanalytic orientation, overemphasize transference and only make transference interventions to group members. For example, given the option of focusing on the relationship between two members or between a member and him- or herself, the therapist may always choose the latter. Or the therapist may always interpret the relationship between two patients only as it pertains to the therapist—e.g., that two members who are being supportive of one another are trying to exclude the therapist, or to arouse jealousy, or to prove they can do without a therapist. If therapists see only the transference aspects of the group, they will fail to encourage the exploration of many other important interactions. They will also fail to relate authentically to many of the group members.

Group therapists must make good use of any irrational or unrealistic attitudes toward themselves without at the same time neglecting their many other functions in the group. To work effectively with transference, therapists must help patients recognize, understand, and change their distorted reactions. There are two major approaches to transference resolution in the therapy group: consensual validation and therapist transparency.

CONSENSUAL VALIDATION

In consensual validation, the therapist encourages a patient to compare his or her impressions of an event in the group with those of other members. For example, if all of the group members concur in a patient's view of the therapist as confrontative and autocratic, then either this patient's reaction to the therapist stems from global group forces related to the leader's role, or the reaction is not unrealistic at all, and the patient is perceiving the therapist quite accurately! Therapists, too, have blind spots.

If, on the other hand, only one member of the group possesses a particular view of the therapist, then this member may be helped to examine the possibility that he or she sees the group therapist, and perhaps other people, too, through an internal, distorting prism. Consensual validation permits patients to recognize the idiosyncratic ways in which they imbue the therapist with characteristics not perceived by other group members.

THERAPIST TRANSPARENCY

Group therapists must learn to respond to their patients authentically, to share their feelings in a judicious and responsible manner, and to acknowledge or refute motives and feelings attributed to them. In other words, they must examine their own blind spots and demonstrate respect for the feedback members offer them. As a clinical example, a contentious male engineering student in a support group for undergraduates accused one of the therapists of being too confrontative and impatient when she asked him to share some reactions with a fellow group member; the therapist had reacted in this fashion, the student asserted, because of feelings of boredom and superiority in the group. In response, the therapist gently reminded this student of his habit of getting into conflict with authority figures, but she also acknowledged that she had often, before, received feedback about her impatience. It was true that she had been feeling restless with the overly careful pace of the group discourse—perhaps she had been excessively active. When therapists demonstrate this kind of personal transparency, it is increasingly difficult for members to maintain their fictitious beliefs or stereotypes about the group leaders.

OBJECTIONS TO THERAPIST TRANSPARENCY

The primary objection to psychotherapist transparency is based on the traditional psychoanalytic belief that the paramount therapeutic factor in psychotherapy is the resolution of patient–therapist transference. In group psychotherapy, however, other therapeutic factors are of equal or greater importance, and the therapist must judiciously use his or her own person in the real-time of the group to encourage the development of these other factors. In modeling interpersonal transparency, the therapist attends to the shaping of norms, and to here-and-now activation and process illumination. By decentralizing his or her position in the group through the use of transparency, the therapist hastens the development of group autonomy and cohesiveness.

Therapists accustomed to maintaining an authoritative position with respect to their patients, especially physicians trained in the medical model, may fear that they will lose power or respect from group members as they disclose their reactions. They may imagine that if they reveal some of themselves their patients will lose faith in them or ridicule them. The therapist who has had some personal group therapy experience recognizes the fallacy of these beliefs.

Another objection therapists raise to personal self-disclosure is the fear of escalation, the fear that once they reveal themselves, the insatiable group will demand even more. Strong forces in the group oppose this trend: Though members are enormously curious about their group leader, they also wish the therapist to remain unknown and all-powerful. While they appreciate the leader's responsible and growth-promoting feedback and personal honesty, few expect or want details of therapists' personal problems.

GUIDELINES TO THE USE OF TRANSPARENCY

There are many different approaches to therapist transparency, depending upon the therapist's personal style and goals in the group at a particular time. An important guideline can be obtained by asking oneself what the purpose of self-disclosure is at any given point in the group—"Am I trying to facilitate transference resolution? Am I model-setting in an effort to create therapeutic norms? Am I attempting to assist the interpersonal learning of members by working on their relationship with me? Am I attempting to support and demonstrate my acceptance of members by saying, in effect, 'I value and respect you and demonstrate this by giving of myself?'" At all times, the therapist must consider whether transparency is consonant with other group therapy tasks.

THERAPIST–PATIENT INTERACTIONS AND TRANSPARENCY

Whenever a therapist–patient interaction occurs, especially one involving feedback from the patient to the therapist, the therapist must be ready to engage in judicious self-disclosure. If, for example, an overly obsequious young anorexic wonders whether the group leader is angry at her for missing a session, the therapist might respond by indicating that, yes, he was worried and, yes, also a little irritated at being given no notice about her absence. He can then go on to explore the repercussions and meaning of his reactions with the patient and the rest of the group: What is it like to hear about his irritation? Is this what the patient expected, or does it seem unreasonable? Was there part of her which hoped to get a rise out of the therapist? How do other group members feel about the patient's absence? Does anyone else in the group have feedback for the leader about his or her reactions?

There are three general principles which the therapist must consider when receiving feedback from group members:

1. The therapist should take the feedback seriously by listening to it, considering it, and responding to it directly.
2. The therapist should obtain consensual validation: How do other members feel? Is the feedback primarily a transference reaction, or does it closely correspond to reality as confirmed by the majority of the group members? If it is reality-based, the therapist must openly confirm this: "Yes, I think you're right in observing how quickly I snapped back at you. Others, too, have noted that I've been irritable this past week."
3. The therapist should measure the feedback against his or her own internal experience: Does the feedback fit? Is there something important to learn from it? The leader who finds herself being told by members that she comes across as somewhat distant and aloof may find that this indeed fits with her feelings in the group; understanding these feelings can provide important lessons for future therapeutic work.

The therapists's role undergoes a gradual metamorphosis during the life of any relatively stable interactional group, and also during many of the more specialized long-term groups (such as a long-term recovery group for alcoholics, or an ongoing support group for intensive care unit nurses). In the beginning, therapists busy themselves with the myriad functions necessary for the creation of the group, and with the development of a social system in which the many therapeutic factors operate. Therapists also devote themselves to the activation and illumination of the here-and-now so that appropriate interpersonal learning can take place. Gradually, however, the therapist goes on to interact with the group as an honest and self-revealing member, and the early stereotypes the patients cast him or her into become more difficult to maintain.

■ USING PROCEDURAL AIDS

A group leader's therapeutic armamentarium can be expanded through the use of procedural aids—specialized techniques that may not be essential, but that may facilitate the course of therapy. These include the use of written summaries, the use of videotaping, and structured exercises. The potential usefulness of these procedural aids depends greatly on the type of therapy group under consideration.

WRITTEN SUMMARIES

The course of most outpatient therapy groups, especially interactionally oriented groups, is facilitated by the use of written summaries (4, 5). The group therapist dictates a candid, concise description of the group session after each meeting, and has a transcription (of approximately two to three single-spaced pages) sent out to the group members the following day. These summaries provide an extra contact with the group between meetings.

AIMS

The summary serves several functions. It provides an understanding of the here-and-now events of the session and facilitates the integration of powerful affective experiences in the group. It labels good or resistant sessions, notes and rewards patient gains in the group, and predicts undesirable developments in the group, thus minimizing their impact. It increases group cohesiveness by emphasizing similarities among members, by underscoring the expression of caring or other positive emotions, and by providing continuity from one meeting to another.

The summary is an ideal forum for interpretations, either for repetition of interpretations made during the session (which may have fallen on deaf ears if delivered in the midst of a melee), or for new interpretations which have occurred to the therapist after the meeting. Summaries are also an additional format for therapist transparency. Most importantly, the summaries provide hope to the patients by helping them realize that the group process is orderly and that the therapists have a coherent sense of the group's long-term development.

GENERAL FEATURES

Although summaries are used only rarely, patients are unanimous in their positive evaluation of this technique. Most await the arrival of the weekly summary in the mail with anticipation; they read and consider it seriously. Many reread the summaries several times and almost all file them for future review. The patient's therapeutic perspective and commitment is deepened; the patient–therapist relationship is strengthened. No serious transference complications, breaks in confidentiality, or other adverse consequences occur.

Weekly summaries must be honest and straightforward about the process of therapy in the group. They are virtually identical to the summaries therapists make for their own files, and are based on the assumption that each patient is a full collaborator in the therapeutic process, that psychotherapy is strengthened and not weakened by demystification. The orientation of the material in the summary reflects the therapeutic orientation of the group. In a long-term interaction group, the summary focuses on the interpersonal transactions that occurred in the meeting and the therapist's reflections on some of the dynamics and implications of those transactions. In a time-limited outpatient group with more modest goals, the focus of the summaries is entirely different. In a group for bereaved spouses, for example, the summaries are more descriptive in nature and underline some of the members' modes of coping with the problems in bereavement: loneliness, change in social role, disposition of the effects of the dead spouse, confrontation with existential issues (death, aloneness, meaning in life, regret). On pages 102-103 are examples of summaries from two different types of groups.

VIDEOTAPING

Some therapists make the videotape recording a central feature of therapy. They arrange for immediate playback of certain segments during a meeting, or set up regularly scheduled playback sessions. Others find the technique valuable, but prefer to use it as a teaching device or occasionally as an auxiliary aid in the therapeutic process (9, 10).

Although feedback from others about one's behavior is important, it is never as convincing as information one discovers for oneself; from this standpoint videotape provides powerful, firsthand feedback. Watching oneself on videotape for the first time is often a significant experience which radically challenges one's self-image. It is not unusual suddenly for patients to recall previ-

(text continued on page 103)

EXAMPLES OF WRITTEN SUMMARIES FROM THERAPY GROUP SESSIONS

I. Bereaved Spouse's Group: time-limited (8 sessions), closed membership

First Session

... After spending some time learning each other's names, we asked members to tell us a little about themselves and what they've been through. We asked people to go only as far as they felt comfortable, and not to open up any memories that feel too painful right now. Janet started the introductions by telling us about herself. She was married for three years and her husband died four months ago of leukemia. She did a lot of nursing care of him and also worked. It was very hard for her after he died. One of her temptations was to seek a new relationship right away ...

... At the end of the meeting, we asked what it was like for members to introduce themselves to the group. Ellen was surprised that she'd been able to talk more in the group than she thought she'd be able to. Bob told us he feels apprehensive about the group because when he talks about his bereavement it dredges up a lot of pain. We discussed briefly the advantages of looking inwardly at our feelings versus trying to distract ourselves. Even though it's painful to look at one's sad feelings too intensely for too long, ultimately it's necessary to explore ourselves fully so we can live with ourselves ...

Eighth Session

This was a very engaged, hard-working meeting with a lot of painful issues being talked about openly. It was also our last meeting and the ending of the group was discussed fully ...

We started by talking about regret and whether people might have regrets about things they wished they had said in the group but did not. This brought up for Janet and Ellen regrets they have at not having communicated as fully as they would have liked with their husbands at the end of their husbands' illness ...

... We examined the question of how to take pressure off of oneself if one feels guilty for something. Ellen talked about how sorry she was that she wasn't more expressive in the group. We pointed out that she had, in fact, started out by finding it difficult to talk in the group. But over the eight weeks she spoke with increasing openness and trust in here. Though she can't alter her past, she's taking this tragic bereavement in her life and attempting to learn from it and to alter her future. Five years from now, she won't have any reason to regret her behavior when she looks back and notes how expressive she has become of her feelings with her children and close friends . . .

II. Long-term Interaction Group: unlimited lifespan, open membership (kept at eight members)

Sixteenth Session

Today's group was intense and honest. It felt like a turning point where deeper issues are beginning to be explored . . .

Alan began by telling the group he had read an article about adult children of alcoholics and was wondering if this kind of organization wouldn't be better for him and whether or not he should leave the group. He received a lot of feedback about this. Sophia noticed how Alan has been getting close to people in the group, and she wondered if he was thinking about leaving because this felt scary to him. Later, when talking about the holidays, Alan mentioned only the good parts. Irv asked if he wasn't obeying an inner injunction to never complain. Alan answered "yes!" and said he learned this as a child. He then was able to share some of the lonely and unsatisfying parts of his holidays. Many members felt real contact with Alan here. Bill said that for the first time, he felt some real empathy with him, and wasn't put off by his "professor-like" manner. Alan worked very hard in the group today and seemed to appreciate the contact he made with other members. We hope this doesn't feel too close or too scary to him when he thinks back on it . . .

Mary was really moving in a new mode today. She took strong stances in the group rather than being in her usual supportive or placating role. Another big change was that she shared some painful memories from her childhood, which we know is difficult for her. Irv pressed her a bit further, and she got in touch with some sad and ashamed feelings. Afterward, Irv and Sophia wondered why these often come up at the end of group when there isn't time left to explore these with her . . .

ous feedback they have gotten from other members. With dramatic impact, they realize that the group has been honest and, if anything, overprotective in previous confrontations.

The therapist's decision to use videotaping as a regular procedural aid depends in great part on the focus and goals of the group at hand. For example, therapists in an intensive group therapy treatment program for patients with functional (somatizing) illness have relied heavily on review of videotaped sessions to foster clearer pictures of self-presentation (11).

In general, patients' initial playback reactions are concerned with physical attractiveness and mannerisms. In subsequent playback sessions, patients begin to make more careful note of their interactions with others, their withdrawal or timidity, their self-preoccupation or aloofness or hostility. Often profound realizations occur: For the first time, patients observe with their own eyes their full behavior and its impact on others.

Patients who are to view the playback are usually receptive to the suggestion of videotaping. Often, however, they are concerned about confidentiality and need reassurance on this issue. If the tape is to be viewed by anyone other than the group members (for example, students, researchers, or supervisors), the therapist must be explicit about the purpose of the viewing and the identity of the viewers and must obtain written permission from all the members.

STRUCTURED EXERCISES

The term structured exercises refers to the many group activities in which the members follow some specific set of orders, generally prescribed by the leader. These kinds of exercises play a more important role in brief, specialized therapy groups than in the long-term general outpatient groups (4, 5, 12).

PURPOSE

The precise rationale for the procedures vary, but, in general, structured exercises are meant to be accelerating devices. Some structured exercises (go-around introductory or warm-up procedures) bypass the hesitant, uneasy first steps of a group. Others speed up interaction by assigning individuals tasks that circumvent cautious, ritualized social behavior (for example, having members in a new group pair up and describe themselves briefly to their partners, then having each member introduce his partner to the whole group). Yet other techniques speed up individual work by helping members to recognize suppressed emotions, or to explore unknown parts of themselves, or to attend to physical sensations. Table 1 contains examples of structured exercises.

TABLE 1. **Examples of Structured Exercises in Psychotherapy Groups**

Members are asked to form dyads. Each person describes him- or herself to the other partner in the dyad for a few minutes. The group reforms. Every member then introduces his or her partner to the group and *speaks for* his or her partner, describing personal characteristics, brief life biography, likes and dislikes, aspirations, etc. Afterward, members explore what it is like to describe oneself in personal detail to another person, and then to have that person share the description with the group. (**Substance abuse group—ongoing recovery**)

Each member in the group is asked to bring in a favorite photograph taken of themselves with at least one other person. During a go-around, each person describes what is special about the photograph while it is passed around the group. Other group members are encouraged to share their reactions. (**Day hospital group**)

Members are given paper and a pencil and asked to write their own obituary. What would they like to be remembered for? What do they consider the true enduring accomplishments of life? Members then read their "obituaries" aloud to the group and give and receive feedback from each other. (**Bereavement group; workshop on death and dying**)

One member of the group ("the questioner") steps out of the meeting room. While he or she is outside, the group selects a person who will be "the subject." The questioner comes back into the room, and attempts to guess the identity of the subject by asking three questions. All three questions must be of the type: "If this person were a _____ (flower, animal, car, or any other category of objects), what kind would he or she be?" Each member, including the subject, must answer each question in turn (for example, "This person would be a tiger lily")— without giving away the identity of the subject! At the end of the go-around of answers to the three questions, the questioner attempts to guess the identity of the subject. The group then discusses how different people's perceptions of the same subject led them to give different answers.

TABLE 1. **Examples of Structured Exercises in Psychotherapy Groups** *(continued)*

Members are asked to think about what kind of mood they are in, and then to use two colors to describe that mood. Each member shares his or her two colors with the group, and the group attempts to deduce the patient's mood and reason for choosing those colors. (**Chronic inpatient group**)

Each member is given seven index cards and a pencil, and is asked to list one personal identifying characteristic on each index card (for example, "I am a teacher" or "I am someone who loves music" or "I am a passionate person"). Members are then instructed to arrange the seven cards so that the most superficial characteristic is on top, the most profound on the bottom. For several minutes, members meditate quietly about giving up the first, most superficial identity. They then move to the next card, then the next, and so on, until they have meditated on giving up even one's most profound identifying characteristics. The process is then repeated in reverse and members re-assume the various identities from most profound to most superficial. The group discusses the thoughts and feelings evoked by the exercise. (**Personal growth group for nonpatients**)

Members are asked to answer the question, "If you had a million dollars, what would you do?" Both humorous answers and more thoughtful replies are required. The group is encouraged to interact around each member's answer. (**Lower-functioning level inpatient group**)

Members are asked to bring in their food diaries and to open them to the page where they describe their most recent episode of bingeing. The diaries are then passed one person to the left. Each member reads her neighbor's entry aloud to the rest of the group and shares her reactions. (**Eating disorders outpatient group**)

An index card and pencil are given to each member. Members anonymously write down one thing they really like about themselves and one thing they would like to change on the card. The cards are put in a pile in the center of the room and mixed. Each member draws a card at random from the pile and reads it aloud. Members then share their reactions to each card. (**Aftercare group**)

A structured exercise may require only a few minutes, or it may consume an entire meeting. Though the exercise may be predominantly verbal or nonverbal in nature, there is always a verbal component in that it generates data that the group subsequently discusses. The exercise may involve the group as a whole—a chronic inpatient group may, for example, be asked to plan an outing. Or it may involve one member vis-a-vis the group—in an encounter-type group, a "trust" exercise involves one member standing, with eyes closed, in the center of the group circle and then falling, allowing the group to support him or her. Exercises can include each individual within the group, such as a go-around where each member is asked to give initial impressions of everyone else in the group. Another type of go-around useful in the early life of a group is to have each member share some background history. In a group for bereaved spouses, members are asked during an early session to bring in a wedding photograph to share with the rest of the group.

Many of the tasks and techniques already described in previous sections—norm-setting, here-and-now activation, understanding the here-and-now—use approaches that have a prescriptive quality. ("Whose opinion in the group especially matters to you?" "Can you look at Mary as you talk to her?" "What has it been like for you to share that with us?" "On a risk-taking scale of 1 to 10, how much have you risked with us today?")

Every experienced group therapist uses some structured exercises, at times in a subtle and spontaneous manner (13). For example, if a group is tense and blocked and experiences a silence of a minute or two (a minute's silence feels very long in a group!), some leaders might ask for a quick go-around in which each member says briefly what he or she has been feeling or has thought of saying, but did not, in that silence. Such an exercise generates much valuable data.

LIMITATIONS

Excessive use of structured exercises is counter-productive. In long-term group therapy, members make more therapeutic headway if the leaders encourage them to experience their timidity or suspiciousness and to understand the underlying dynamics rather than prescribing an exercise which circumvents those feelings by plunging members into deep disclosure or expressivity.

In acute or short-term settings, such as inpatient groups and certain specialized outpatient groups, the situation is more complex. Faced with a limited amount of time in which to be helpful to many different patients, therapists may find that structured exercises are extremely useful: they increase patient participation, provide a discrete, appropriate group task, and increase the group efficiency. But there is a pitfall to be avoided. Whenever therapists make heavy use of structured tasks, they run the risk of creating a dependent group. Norms are established in which most of the activity and interactions in the group are generated through the directions of the leader, rather than through the active and motivated participation of the members. Patients in a highly structured, therapist-centered group begin to feel that help, all help, emanates from the therapist alone. They do not allow their skills to develop and they cease to avail themselves of the help and resources that other group members can provide. The therapist must therefore tread a fine line between energizing and infantilizing the group.

■ REFERENCES

1. Lieberman MA: Change induction in small groups. Ann Rev Psychol 1976; 27:217-250
2. Kahn EM: Group treatment interventions for schizophrenics. Int J Group Psychother 1984; 34:149-153
3. Rothke S: The role of interpersonal feedback in group therapy. Int J Group Psychother 1986; 36:225-240
4. Yalom ID: The Theory and Practice of Group Psychotherapy. New York, Basic Books, 1970
5. Yalom ID: The Theory and Practice of Group Psychotherapy, 3rd ed. New York, Basic Books, 1985
6. Bion WR: Experiences in groups and other papers. New York, Basic Books, 1959
7. Nichols M, Taylor T: Impact of therapist interventions on early sessions of group therapy. J Clin Psychol 1975; 31:726-729
8. Malan D: Group psychotherapy: a long term follow-up study. Arch Gen Psychiatry 1976; 33:1303-1315
9. Berger M: The use of videotape in the integrated treatment of individuals, couples, families and groups in private practice, in Videotape Techniques in Psychiatric Training and Treatment. Edited by Berger M. New York, Brunner/Mazel, 1970

10. Rynearson EK, Flanagan P: Distortions of self-image and audio-visual therapy. Psychiatric Annals 1982; 12:1082-1085
11. Melson SJ, Rynearson EK: Intensive group therapy for functional illness. Psychiatric Annals 1986; 16:687-692
12. Lieberman MA, Yalom ID, Miles MB: Encounter Groups: First Facts. New York, Basic Books, 1973
13. Corey G, Corey MS, Callanan P, et al: Group Techniques. Monterey, CA, Brooks/Cole Publishing Co., 1982

INPATIENT GROUPS   7

Any attempt to classify the vast array of specialized groups in current clinical practice would begin with the line of cleavage between inpatient and outpatient settings. The general category of inpatient groups can be further subdivided according to level of acuity (Figure 1). Acute inpatient groups, such as those that meet on psychiatric wards in general hospitals, have many complex features that have been described throughout this book (Table 1). They are different in nature from the chronic inpatient groups one encounters in a Veterans Administration hospital or in a long-term psychiatric care facility for the chronic mentally ill. These latter groups show greater resemblance to aftercare and medication clinic groups in the outpatient setting.

Although we have placed outpatient groups at the pole opposite from inpatient groups, therapists working with certain kinds of specialized inpatient groups will encounter many of the same clinical situations, and will utilize many of the same techniques, as their colleagues in the outpatient setting (the reader is referred to the corresponding sections on specialized outpatient groups). After all, a behaviorally oriented group for patients with anorexia nervosa held on a medical-psychiatric ward has a greater number of similarities to, than differences from, the same sort of group held in an eating disorders clinic.

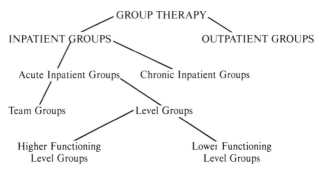

FIGURE 1. **Classificatory Scheme for Specialized Psychotherapy Groups**

TABLE 1. **Features of Inpatient Psychotherapy Groups**

- Rapid changes in group composition
- Patients undergoing a brief hospitalization only participate in group for a few sessions
- Frequent meetings (often daily)
- Little or no pre-group preparation
- Presence of severe psychopathology
- Great heterogeneity in patients' psychopathology
- Rotating staff/lack of continuity in group leaders
- Myriad effects of ward milieu on group process
- Presence of extra-group socializing
- May be only form of psychotherapy available to patient
- May be only forum to address stress of hospitalization

■ ACUTE INPATIENT GROUPS

In order to modify general group psychotherapy techniques to suit any specialized setting, whether it might be an acute inpatient group or a long-term recovery group for alcoholics, the therapist must follow three steps:

1. *Assess the clinical situation:* The therapist must determine the mutable and immutable clinical restraints surrounding the group he or she wishes to lead. They must attempt to alter the mutable restraints in a direction favorable for their group.
2. *Formulate goals:* The therapist must develop goals that are appropriate and achievable within the existing clinical restraints.
3. *Modify traditional technique:* The therapist must retain the basic principles of group therapy, but alter techniques to adapt to the clinical setting and to achieve the specified goals.

In this section, we shall illustrate these three steps as they are applied to the acute inpatient therapy group (1). Such groups occur on adult general psychiatric units and involve a wide range of patients undergoing acute hospitalization for an almost infinite array of problems, from suicidality to psychosis to behavioral dyscontrol. Radical modifications of technique are required in order to lead effective groups in the inpatient setting.

ASSESSING THE CLINICAL SITUATION

The therapist must start with a thorough assessment of the clinical setting, determining which of the constraints facing him or her are intrinsic to the clinical situation, and therefore beyond control, and which are extrinsic and potentially modifiable.

Intrinsic limitations to the acute inpatient setting—over which the therapist has no control—include the rapid turnover of patients (patients often will be present for only a single group meeting!) and the severity and heterogeneity of psychopathology among hospitalized patients. In addition, the rotation of staff on inpatient units often precludes continuity in group leadership (Table 1).

Extrinsic constraints stem from lack of administrative support for group therapy: For example, the ward policy may be to schedule groups once or twice a week for brief periods, to have no permanent group therapist, to assign inexperienced staff as leaders, or to take patients out of group. The job of the therapist who is designing an inpatient group begins with a campaign for the best possible conditions. The support of administrative and clinical staff must be enlisted to ensure that group therapy is an integral part of the ward program, that group time is set aside and protected for all patients, and that there are adequate group meeting room facilities. Program directors must be persuaded of the efficacy and importance of group therapy, using, if necessary, available research findings.

A third factor that influences inpatient group therapy is the ward milieu, the larger ecosystem in which the group is nestled. Parallel processes occur throughout the system, and stress within the ward—either among patients, among patients and staff, or among staff members—will boomerang back into the group. For example, an internecine struggle between two nurses competing for an administrative position may suddenly be mirrored in strife erupting between two dominant members in the inpatient therapy group.

FORMULATING SPECIFIC GOALS

Once the therapist has arranged the best possible conditions (such as a suitable meeting room, sufficient protected group time, consistency of leaders, some control over group composition), he or she must proceed to formulate appropriate goals for the group. These goals must be specific, achievable in the time frame of the group, and tailored to the capacities of the patients so that group therapy is a success experience (Table 2).

Six achievable goals for the inpatient group as described by Yalom (1) are:

1. Engaging the patient in the therapeutic process: helping the patient to become involved in a process that he or she finds constructive and supportive and will wish to continue after discharge from the hospital. For some patients, hospitalization is their first contact with psychotherapy.

TABLE 2. **Modifying General Group Psychotherapy Techniques for the Acute Inpatient Group**

---

1. Assess the clinical situation: see Table 1

2. Formulate appropriate goals:

- Engage patient in therapeutic process
- Teach patients that talking helps
- Teach problems to problem-spot maladaptive interpersonal behavior
- Decrease patients' sense of isolation
- Allow patients to be helpful to others
- Alleviate hospital-related anxiety

3. Modify general techniques to suit the inpatient setting:

- Adopt an altered time frame
- Use direct support
- Emphasize the here-and-now
- Provide structure

---

2. Teaching patients that talking helps, and that they may use psychotherapy for their benefit.
3. Problem-spotting: helping patients learn to identify their maladaptive interpersonal behavior. In this way, patients identify areas that they can work on in later therapy. Rich data are available from inpatient group psychotherapy, but there is little time to explore these data fully.
4. Decreasing patients' sense of isolation, both in the hospital, and in their outside life.
5. Allowing patients to be helpful to others. Patients entering the hospital are demoralized and gain a great deal from learning they can be of value to others.
6. Alleviating hospital-related anxiety: encouraging patients to share concerns about the stigma of psychiatric hospitalization, to discuss distressing events on the ward (bizarre behavior of other patients, staff tensions, acutely disturbed patients), and to be reassured by other group members.

MODIFYING GENERAL TECHNIQUES TO ACHIEVE SPECIFIC GOALS

Once appropriate goals have been established, therapists must modify standard techniques in order to achieve those specific goals. This means that therapists will vary their basic strategy and tactics in their use of the different therapeutic factors. For example, a therapist may choose to emphasize universality and imparting information in a group of chronic psychotic patients, but, as we shall describe, will emphasize altruism, cohesiveness, and interpersonal learning in an acute inpatient group.

Acute inpatient groups are radically different from traditional long-term outpatient groups (Table 1). They thus require a radical modification in technique, particularly in the areas of time frame, degree of support, use of here-and-now activation, and structure.

THE ALTERED TIME FRAME

The inpatient group leader must adopt a radically shortened time frame because of rapid membership turnover and the fact that group composition changes daily. Therapists must consider the life of an inpatient group to be only a single session, and they must strive to offer something useful for as many patients as possible during that session.

A single-session time frame demands efficiency. There is no time to waste: The leader has only a single opportunity to engage each patient, and must not squander it. This need for efficiency demands heightened therapist activity. The therapist must be prepared to activate the group, to call on members, to support them, and to interact personally with them.

SUPPORT

In order to achieve the goals of creating a constructive, safe, and positive experience with inpatient group therapy, the leader must minimize conflict and emphasize support. Because of the nature of the altered time frame, and because of the high level of distress and the acute sense of crisis experienced by inpatients, the inpatient group therapist must offer support quickly and directly. The most direct manner is simply to acknowledge openly each patient's efforts, intentions, strengths, positive contributions, and risks.

If, for example, a member states that he finds a woman in the group very attractive, the leader must judiciously support this patient for the risk he has taken. The leader may wonder whether he has previously been able to express his admiration of another person so openly, or may note that his openness encourages other members to take risks and reveal important feelings. Positive rather than negative aspects of a person's behavior or defense must be emphasized. For example, the patient who insists on playing "assistant therapist" can be offered positive comments about how helpful this has been to others; the stage is then set for a gentle remark on his or her selflessness and reluctance to ask for something personal from the group.

The actively supportive inpatient therapist makes a specific point of helping patients—especially objectionable or irritating patients—obtain support from the group. A self-absorbed patient who incessantly complains about a health condition, or an insoluble situational problem, will quickly alienate any group. When therapists identify such behavior, they must intervene quickly to circumvent the development of group animosity and rejection. They may, for example, assign the patient the task of introducing new members into the group, or of giving feedback to other members, or of attempting to guess and express what each member's evaluation of the group is that day.

The therapist may also reframe a patient's irritating behavior: "Perhaps you have needs, too, but have trouble asking for what you need. I wonder if your preoccupation with your health (or your finances, or your husband, or the like) isn't a way of asking for something from the group." Helping the patient to formulate an explicit, specific request for attention from the group will often generate a positive response from the other members.

The therapist must anticipate and avoid confrontation and conflict whenever possible. If patients are irritable or critical, therapists can channel some of the anger towards themselves ("Several people seem annoyed in today's session. Is there something I could be doing differently?") If two patients are locked in an adversarial position, the leader can remind them that sparks often fly between two people who are similar, or who have envious feelings toward each other. Then each of the patients can be invited to talk about those aspects of the other that they admire or envy, or to discuss the ways that they resemble their adversary.

When therapists lead a group of severely regressed patients, they must provide even more support and in an even more direct fashion. The patients' behavior must be reframed in some positive way. A mute patient, for example, can be thanked for staying the whole session; the patient who leaves early can be complimented for having stayed even 20 minutes; inactive patients can be supported for having paid attention throughout the meeting. Inappropriate or bizarre statements by patients should be labeled as attempts to communicate with the group, and the group focus should then be gently redirected away from the deviant patient.

EMPHASIZING THE HERE-AND-NOW

These foregoing considerations of therapist efficiency, activity, and support in the inpatient setting do not make the here-and-now focus any less important than it is in outpatient therapy. The here-and-now focus can help inpatients learn many important interpersonal skills:

1. to communicate more clearly
2. to get closer to others
3. to express positive feelings
4. to become aware of personal mannerisms that push people away
5. to listen
6. to offer support
7. to reveal oneself
8. to form friendships

However, the clinical conditions of the inpatient group (brief treatment duration and more severe pathology) demand here-and-now modifications in basic technique. There is insufficient time to work through interpersonal issues. Instead, the therapist helps patients to spot major interpersonal problems and to reinforce interpersonal strengths. This kind of interactional problem-spotting and positive reinforcement occurs within the context of a single group session, and this principle should be made clear to the patients.

PROVIDING STRUCTURE

Work with the acute inpatient group requires structure; there is no place in acute inpatient group work for the nondirective therapist or for the unstructured, free-flowing group.

Group leaders provide structure for the inpatient group in several ways:

1. by instructing and orienting patients as to the nature and purpose of the meeting
2. by establishing very clear spatial and temporal boundaries for the group
3. by using a lucid and confident personal style that reassures confused or anxious patients and contributes to a sense of structure.

The most potent and explicit way of providing structure in the inpatient setting is to build into each session a consistent sequence of events. Although different inpatient group sessions will have different sequences depending on the composition and task of the group, the following are natural lines of cleavage:

1. The first few minutes: The therapist explicitly describes the structure of the group. If there are new members (and there usually are in the acute inpatient group), this is the time to orient them to the purpose of group therapy. Explicit instruction must be provided about the relevance of the here-and-now, by, for example, explaining that group psychotherapy focuses upon the way people relate to one another because that is what groups do best. The therapist can then proceed to explain that groups do this most effectively by examining the relationships among members of the group. The group therapist must emphasize that, though patients may enter the hospital for many different reasons, everyone can benefit from learning how to get more out of their relationships with others.

2. Definition of the task: The therapist determines the most profitable direction for the group to take in a particular session. The leader may, for example, listen to get a sense of the urgent issues present on the ward that day—a patient who has eloped, or the presence of a new rotation of residents and medical students.

The leader may choose to provide a structured exercise, such as helping each patient formulate an agenda that he or she wants to work on during that session (1). An example of an "agenda" might be the shy and inhibited young depressed woman who would like to try and express some positive feelings in the group.

3. Accomplishing the task: The therapist helps the group address the issues or agendas raised at the start of the session and encourages as many patients to participate as possible. Each group member is asked about what his or her reaction was to the patient who eloped; the shy patient is helped to identify the members she feels positively toward and to express those feelings.

4. The final few minutes: The leader indicates that the work phase is over and the remaining time is devoted to reviewing and analyzing the meeting. This is the summing up period and the self-reflective loop of the here-and-now in which the therapist attempts to clarify the group interaction that occurred in the session. How, for example, did the group respond when a usually quiet and inhibited member openly expressed some positive sentiments? What was it like to talk openly about a patient's elopement?

WORKING WITHIN THE WARD MILIEU

Regulation of the semipermeable boundaries that exist between the inpatient group and the ward milieu is also an important task of the inpatient group therapist. This is accomplished by establishing clear contracts between patients and staff (as part of the explicit ward rules or expectations for behavior) and within the group itself regarding the basic boundaries listed in Table 3 (2).

When the group task and the limits surrounding that task are defined clearly and explicitly in this manner, the inpatient group will appear less fragmented and more stable, and it will be able to maintain its integrity within the larger ward environment. Furthermore, vulnerable prepsychotic and psychotic patients are protected from experiencing personal boundary diffusion.

Without a sense of group cohesion in the ever-changing environment of the ward milieu, therapy cannot take place. Punctuality, predictability, high expectations for attendance and performance, and daily meetings to minimize massive group composition changes all contribute to group cohesion. In addition, as

TABLE 3 **Basic Boundaries for the Inpatient Therapy Group in the Ward Milieu**

- Clear contracts about punctuality and attendance for patients participating in group

- Beginning and ending each group meeting on time

- Safeguarding group time on the ward (not scheduling activities which interfere with group time)

- Protecting patients' time in the group (not permitting patients to miss group sessions for other activities)

- Clear criteria for patient entry and participation in the group and for patient exit from the group

- Firm limits for excluding incompatible patients from group sessions

- Strict norms for acceptable behavior in the group

- Instruction about confidentiality of topics discussed in group

described in another section, clarifying the rationale and goals of the group, and orienting patients explicitly to these goals, either prior to entry into the group or at the beginning of each meeting, increases group cohesion in the midst of the ward milieu (3).

Finally, therapists must recall that dynamics and processes occurring in the acute inpatient group are often reflected back onto other interactions on the ward, and vice versa:

A manipulative transsexual patient often exploded angrily during group sessions on an inpatient unit, intimidating the other members with his discussions of sexual identity, and insisting that he be addressed with a feminine pronoun. The group's fear and confusion was reflected in the milieu's response to the patient: Very experienced staff members began complying with the patient's unreasonable demands, including assignment to a private room, unusual day passes to attend electrolysis sessions, and histrionic outbursts that would have been rapidly controlled in any other patient.

The group leader, a second-year resident, was finally able to set limits on the patient's subtly threatening behavior in group—

but only after her attending psychiatrist spoke up during a staff meeting and pointed out the many ways in which this patient was holding the entire ward hostage to his angry, self-centered demands. This example demonstrates that the group therapist on an inpatient unit must work closely with staff to identify the dynamics occurring in the lilieu that are influencing interactions in the group and vice versa.

GROUP COMPOSITION

The patient population of acute inpatient wards is highly heterogeneous both in terms of formal diagnosis and overall level of ego-strength and functioning. If any similarity or homogeneity exists among inpatients, it is that they have entered the hospital in crisis, are experiencing a high degree of psychological distress and vulnerability, and are facing a major disruption of their everyday lives and activities. Even though they are all greatly distressed, inpatients may have such disparate levels of functioning that they are not all able to work in the same kind of therapy group.

Given the vastly different therapeutic needs of a hallucinating, paranoid schizophrenic experiencing her fourth psychotic episode and a recently widowed professional hospitalized for the first time with major depression, it is clear that a single group composed heterogeneously of all the patients in an acute inpatient ward may not be able to address all of the goals appropriate for the various members. And yet, if patients are to be separated into different sorts of groups, on what basis should the triage occur?

Yalom addresses the question of group composition in his comprehensive model of inpatient group psychotherapy (1). He suggests that patients be offered two kinds of group experiences on the ward: a team group for all patients regardless of diagnosis or level of functioning (which consists of a daily, mandatory, heterogeneously composed group of approximately 6 to 10 members), and a level group determined by level of functioning.

As an example of a team group, the patient population on a 20-bed unit is randomly divided equally between 2 small groups, each led by a nurse and one of the psychiatric residents on the unit. These small, heterogeneous groups meet early in the day, are content-oriented, and deal with external problems, including major milieu issues, and the welcoming or leave-taking of patients. The purpose of these groups is to provide a safe, non-intense, non-interpersonally oriented format where problem-sharing, advice-giving, and support can occur among all patients. It is mandatory for every patient on the ward, with the exception of severely disruptive individuals (such as acutely manic patients); it thus mixes people from different diagnostic categories and allows for all the patients to meet and interact with one another. It also involves every patient on the ward in a group experience, even those who might a priori be resistant to participating in group therapy.

The second type of group, the level group, consists of homogeneous groups geared toward level of ego-strength and overall functioning. After all, different kinds of inpatients will need and value different aspects of group therapy. Patients diagnosed with depressive reaction have been reported to value most highly a group which problem-solves and encourages a focus on external concerns, while schizophrenic patients were shown to prefer non-verbal, activity-oriented groups (4). Even the same patient may be able to progress through various treatment approaches, and utilize different sorts of groups over the length of a relatively short hospitalization. The basic features of team groups versus level groups are outlined in Table 4.

LEVEL GROUPS FOR LOWER-FUNCTIONING PATIENTS

In a level group for lower-functioning patients, the more regressed, withdrawn, or disorganized patients participate in a brief (45 minutes) highly structured activity-oriented group session. The goals of lower-functioning level groups are to encourage reality contact through accurate perception of the immediate environment, and to foster improved ego functioning. A variety of daily living skills and basic socialization issues are often addressed, including budget planning, shopping, learning how to initiate and carry on a simple conversation, and how to handle a job interview. Didactic education may at times be used by the group leaders.

In a typical group session, attendance is mandatory; the leader begins by having members introduce themselves. The leader then presents the topic or group task for that session—for example, by informing the group that today members are going to

TABLE 4. **Features of Inpatient Team Groups and Inpatient Level Groups**

Team Groups	Level Groups
All patients participate	Some patients participate
Mandatory attendance	Usually voluntary, contractual attendance
Patients randomly assigned to group, evenly divided between groups	Patients assigned to group based on level of functioning
Meet early in day	Meet later in day
Meet daily	Meet 3–4 times per week
Led by rotating ward clinicians (psychiatric residents, therapists assigned to the team, etc.)	Led by more stable, trained therapists; attempt to have more continuity in leadership
Deal with content-oriented, external issues	Foster interpersonal engagement in a manner appropriate to level of functioning of patients

learn about enhancing self-esteem. Specific instructions are given for this task, such as requesting that each member in turn tell the group about a personal quality of which he or she is proud. Supportive, positive feedback is then explicitly solicited for each member: "Nina just told us that she is proud of her ability to make friends quickly. Marge, what do you think it is about Nina that makes her so friendly?" If Marge answers in an inappropriate or hostile manner ("Nina makes friends, but often it's because she wants something from them"), the therapist moves in quickly to defuse the situation, without attempting to have the group understand why Marge is giving Nina this feedback: "It seems like Marge too has noticed that Nina makes friends pretty easily. That's a quality we'd all like to have."

Groups for lower-functioning patients are thus very content-oriented, with little commentary on the interactions among members. Leaders must monitor the level of anxiety in the group closely to prevent interpersonal and sensory overstimulation (for example, by switching the focus away from Nina if it appears that there is an argument brewing). Maladaptive behavior both in and outside the group is identified, addressed, and discouraged. ("Marge, you said something positive to Nina, but then you took it away. Today let's just work on positive feedback. Could you try again to comment on Nina's friendliness?")

Yalom describes an interactional group format tailored specifically to lower-functioning patients, entitled Focus Group. Safe, supportive, nonintense interpersonal engagement is fostered through careful leader direction and an organized format that makes use of structured exercises. Typical exercises relate to six main areas: self-disclosure, empathy, here-and-now interaction, didactic discussion, personal change, and tension-alleviating games (see Table 5). The therapist regulates the intensity of interactions occurring in the group by altering members' attention to the content/process ratio, according to the ego-strength and functional capacity of the group as a whole.

TABLE 5. **Examples of Structured Exercise from Lower-Functioning Groups (Focus Groups)**

1. Self-disclosure:
Members are asked to complete one or more brief, focused sentences that require some safe self-disclosure around a given topic. Examples include:
"One of my favorite hobbies is _____."
"The last time I got really angry was when _____."
"One of my best accomplishments is _____."
"When Jim threatened to hurt someone on the ward yesterday, I felt _____."
Members may be asked to pair up into dyads and share their answers. The group then re-forms, and members read aloud their answers or their partners' answers. The group is encouraged to share reactions to each member's answers.

2. Empathy:
A collection of magazine pictures is placed in the center of the room. Members are asked to choose two pictures which they think the person sitting on their left will like. Members then, in turn, show the pictures they chose to the group and explain why they thought the person to their left would like them.

TABLE 5. **Examples of Structured Exercise from Lower-Functioning Groups (Focus Groups)** *(continued)*

---

3. Here-and-now interaction:

Members are asked to pair up. They are then asked to "find two ways in which you are alike, and find two ways in which you are different." Each pair is then asked to share their findings with the rest of the group.

4. Didactic instruction:

The therapist leads a brief, focused discussion on a topic of interest to the group (anger, tension, communication skills). The discussion may be combined with, or preceded by, a specific task: "Please write down three things that are important for good communication between people."

5. Personal change:

Members are asked to complete two sentences:
"A change I want to make in myself is _____."
"One idea I have about how to start making this change is _____."

Members then pair up, share their answers, and come up with additional suggestions for how to start making these changes. The group re-forms, and members present each other's answers and ask for additional suggestions from the group.

6. Tension-relieving games:

Members are asked to observe each other carefully for a few minutes. One designated member of the group is then asked to leave the room briefly while another member in the room slightly alters his or her appearance (takes off some glasses, or exchanges jewelry with another member, or rolls up sleeves, etc.) The designated member returns to the room and attempts to spot the change.

The process of encouraging interpersonal interaction through prescribed and indirect, content-oriented means rather than through a direct, process-oriented manner, is the hallmark of lower-functioning level groups. Such groups are targeted to psychotic patients with impaired reality testing. This approach protects vulnerable patients from an interpersonal intimacy that would be both frightening and fragmenting, and that could aggravate their propensity to withdraw or to retreat into regressed behavior.

Homogeneous inpatient groups geared to individuals with impaired ego functioning are the groups of choice in the treatment of patients with chronic psychotic illness. Such patients generally do poorly in heterogeneous inpatient groups, and in community meetings they are unable to perform the group task and are considered disruptive by other members. This aggravates the psychotic patient's already exquisite sense of estrangement and isolation, and the group becomes another failure experience. However, in a group format where specific tasks are targeted to the lower-functioning patient—such as learning other patients' names, performing nonthreatening structured exercises, discussing medication effects and problems in daily living—and where positive interpersonal interactions are a happy coincidence of the task, the group experience is one of success (5).

LEVEL GROUPS FOR HIGHER-FUNCTIONING PATIENTS

Level groups for higher-functioning patients are designed to facilitate patient interaction and interpersonal learning in the here-and-now microcosm of the inpatient group. They are for nonpsychotic patients who can tolerate the interpersonal intensity and stimulation of a process-oriented group, and who have the necessary concentration and attention to participate in such a group session. A model for a high-functioning acute inpatient group is the Agenda Group (1).

The leader begins the Agenda Group by helping each patient to formulate an interpersonal agenda that he or she would like to address in that particular session. If a patient offers an agenda such as, "I want to be more in touch with my feelings," the therapist begins to shape it by wondering, "Adam, how can we help you be in touch with your feelings in group today? Is there some way we can make it easier for you to share your feelings with us here in the group this afternoon?" Each agenda must be shaped into a personal, specific, here-and-now concern that can be addressed face-to-face in the group session with the assistance of the other members (see Table 6 for examples of agendas).

The round of agendas takes approximately 30 minutes, or approximately one-third of the group time. Agendas force vague complaints and concerns to become specific and to be stated aloud in a clear, coherent manner. Patients are forced to take

TABLE 6. **Examples of Interpersonal Agendas from Higher-Functioning Level Groups (Agenda Groups)**

1. *Patient*: "I would like a clearer picture of how I come across to others."

   Therapist: "Would you be willing to accept some feedback from people here in the group today about how you come across to them? From whom here in the room would you especially like such feedback? Why do you want to get a clearer picture of how others see you?"

2. *Patient*: "I would like to express some feelings and not hold everything inside."

   Therapist: "What kinds of feelings would you like to try and express today to us here in the group? Would you be willing to express such feelings as they come up in today's meeting? Can we check in with you from time to time to see what kinds of feelings you're having during the session?"

3. *Patient*: "I want to learn to be more assertive."

   Therapist: "Would you be willing to try and assert yourself here in the group today? Would you like to try and ask for something for yourself, like how much time you'd like in the group? Would you try to say one thing you would ordinarily hold back?"

4. *Patient*: "I want to feel less lonely and isolated from people."

   Therapist: "From whom do you feel isolated here in the group? Would you be willing to explore the ways you avoid getting close to people? Would you like to try a different way of approaching people here in the group today? Would you like feedback from us on how you create distance?"

---

responsibility for their work in the group session, and the tendency to engage in wasteful small talk, story-telling, and silences is reduced.

After the agenda go-around, the leader spends the next 30-45 minutes in helping members fill each other's agenda, using an explicit here-and-now focus. "Adam, Rob just told us about his recent divorce. Your agenda is to share some of your feelings in here with us today. What are Rob's comments stirring up for you?" Or, better yet (to the group as a whole), "Rob just told us about his painful divorce. Is there some way we could make this helpful for Adam's agenda?" The here-and-now focus enhances immediate group interaction because each patient has stated an agenda that must be worked on, in the group session, with the aid of the other members. This centripetal force of the group task allows a number of different patient agendas to be worked on simultaneously.

The leader ends each meeting with a review that takes place in the group room, in front of the group participants. Co-therapists and any observers (students, residents, mental health trainees, ward staff) who have watched the group take part in this review. The leaders openly discuss their interventions and the success of each member's agenda, actively supporting the patients' therapeutic efforts; observers provide feedback on this process. "I found that Adam really shared some sadness with us today after we asked him how he felt about Rob's story ... I liked how Sue told Adam it made him seem more human and less distant from the rest of us." Or, "While we were observing you through the two-way mirror, we found ourselves wondering why you stepped in and asked about Adam, when it seemed that Mary was the one having a really strong reaction to Rob's story."

Agenda group members observe the therapists reviewing the session, and the effect is threefold:

1. It demystifies the process of psychotherapy.
2. It provides cognitive structure and thus destimulates members prior to leaving the meeting.
3. It helps to make each meeting as self-contained as possible— the time frame of the group becomes reduced to a single meeting, which helps to minimize the effects of daily compositional changes.

Here-and-now techniques are often avoided in acute inpatient group therapy, perhaps because they are mistakenly equated with confrontation and conflict. In fact, this approach is a highly supportive and validating experience, especially for patients who are overwhelmed by feelings of helplessness, isolation, and disengagement. The stimulation of interpersonal learning occurring in a positive and therapeutic manner gives patients a sense of mastery over their own behavior, and, through the mechanism of altruism, allows them to feel helpful to others. If there is any caveat to be made, it is simply that, as with lower-functioning groups, the therapist will need to remain alert to potentially volatile and angry situations, and when they occur, will need to act quickly to defuse them.

■ CHRONIC INPATIENT GROUPS

The clinician working in a large institution such as a Veterans Administration hospital, a correctional facility, or a public sector mental hospital may find him- or herself confronted with inpatient groups where members remain in the treatment setting for several weeks or months.

Chronic inpatient groups show a mixture of features. On the one hand, some of their clinical constraints are similar to those we have already described for acute inpatient groups, including the fact that the milieu is all-pervasive, that extra-group socializing occurs, that the patient is suffering from severe problems that necessitated institutionalization, and that groups meet regularly and frequently and are sometimes the only forum to address the stresses of being in the hospital (Table 1). In contrast to acute inpatient groups, however, the patient population is more stable on a chronic inpatient ward, and therefore both group composition and milieu composition show a certain predictability and continuity.

CLINICAL SITUATION AND GOALS

Group psychotherapy has been used for chronic inpatients since the 1920s, and research over the years has documented its efficacy in reducing the psychological morbidity for these patients. Although the advent of antipsychotic medication has changed the clinical picture of psychotic illness, research indicates that group psychotherapy and pharmacotherapy reinforce one another: a higher success rate in the treatment of schizophrenia has been observed when group therapy is combined with pharmacotherapy (6). In another study, schizophrenics who received group psychotherapy plus antipsychotic medication showed greater improvement in social effectiveness and behavior and were rehospitalized significantly less often after a two-year period than were those receiving medication plus individual psychotherapy (7). In other words, medication does not replace group therapy for the chronic mentally ill.

If group treatment of schizophrenic patients is difficult, it is because of certain intrinsic clinical considerations rather than because of the group modality. For example, psychotic patients are often actively hallucinating, paranoid, disorganized, mute, or withdrawn from others. They often suffer from overwhelming fear and distrust (8, 9). Extrinsic constraints to chronic inpatient group psychotherapy include problems with staffing therapy groups (such as problems with understaffing), and the unwillingness of staff to devote time to group treatment.

There are several difficulties that occur in leading chronic inpatient groups:

1. Hostility and ambivalence toward the leader is great because of paranoid ideation and an inability to differentiate between the leader and other authority figures.
2. The group has severe problems developing autonomy and cohesiveness.
3. Communication is inhibited and distorted among the chronic mentally ill.

Cohesiveness and autonomy are extremely difficult to achieve in such groups because members often resent participation and devalue the group. They also show great dependence on the leader, and are more susceptible to therapist approval than to group pressure. Group standards almost never are adhered to automatically—they require repeated confirmation by the leader.

Communication is limited and often distorted among the chronic mentally ill. The comments of individual members are frequently autistic in nature, and may not possess a common theme or even relate to a group event. The monopolist patient is common and is managed poorly by members. Suicidal ideation and existential despair occur often and become contagious. In these and other crises, members withdraw from one another, or act impulsively and destructively. Patients project their own intrapsychic conflict onto the group and do not accept interpretations about group behavior.

These difficult clinical considerations notwithstanding, therapists must remember that the group provides the only real, continuous, consistent social experience for the majority of its members. These patients must live together for long periods of time under confining and stressful circumstances; group psychotherapy can, if done well, reduce some of the day-to-day friction that results, while gratifying patients' emotional needs for friendship and interpersonal relating. The therapeutic factors of universality, altruism, imitative behavior, and socializing techniques are particularly salient in working with this population. Goals of the groups include:

1. learning to relate better to others
2. learning to cope more effectively with problems such as impulse control, auditory hallucinations, and suspicions
3. sharing information about medications, housing, and treatment facilities
4. planning discharge

TASKS AND TECHNIQUES

Chronic inpatient therapy groups should consist of four to eight members. Groups of nine or more are difficult to manage, particularly when patients are severely disruptive or show agitated behavior. Attendance must be mandatory, and participation can be augmented through the use of coffee and snacks as an additional reward for attendance.

During each session, especially if there is a new patient, the goals and rules of the group must be repeated and reinforced by asking one or two of the more experienced members to summarize them. This reminds members of the group norms, and focuses the session on relevant issues. It also lets new members learn that it is permissible to discuss topics such as hearing voices or believing that a nefarious plot exists. This enhances group cohesiveness by showing new patients that they are not alone in having psychotic symptoms. Group rules that should be reinforced actively at each session are listed in Table 7.

TABLE 7.   **Rules of Behavior for Chronic Inpatient Groups**

- Patients must arrive on time

- Patients must stay for the whole session

- Shouting or threatening behavior is not permitted

- Patients must not be destructive of furniture or other objects in the meeting room

---

Therapists must be even more active, supportive, and flexible when working with these chronic patients than they are in the acute inpatient setting. They must encourage interactions among patients clearly and directly—especially helpful and altruistic interactions ("Kevin, could you tell Mickey about how to go and get a special bus pass?"). Whenever possible, gentle here-and-now interactions can be fostered ("Allison, who offered helpful advice today about the residential treatment center?").

At times, leaders can make judicious use of therapist transparency. This will serve as role-modeling, and will encourage imitative behavior: "Moving to a new place is always hard—I know that for me, asking a lot of questions and finding some new friends makes being in a new place easier." Therapist directness and honesty also aids patients to test reality and to correct distorted transference reactions: "No, I do not have a hidden tape recorder in here to report back to the VA police. I am here as your doctor, and I keep the group meeting confidential."

A patient may begin responding to delusions or hallucinations during the group session; the leader must intervene immediately and, if possible, ask other members to provide feedback and guidance to the psychotic individual. Another common difficulty is monopolization by a patient with more affective (often manic) features; such a patient will talk circles around the group, intimidating shy, introverted schizophrenic patients. If they become too disruptive, such patients must simply be withdrawn from the session.

In sum, chronic inpatient groups must be geared to be socially supportive and nonthreatening. The therapist's work will occur in three major arenas:

1. encouraging member-to-member interactions in any way possible
2. fostering altruistic acts
3. stepping in skillfully and forcefully to control disruptive behavior

Challenging as they may be, chronic inpatient groups can go far in improving the quality of day-to-day life on the long-term psychiatric ward and in preparing patients for aftercare once they are discharged (10–12).

■ REFERENCES

1. Yalom ID: Inpatient Group Psychotherapy. New York, Basic Books, 1983
2. Leszcz M: Inpatient groups, in American Psychiatric Association Annual Review, Vol. 5. Edited by Frances AJ, Hales RE. Washington, DC, American Psychiatric Press, Inc., 1986
3. Maxmen JS: Helping patients survive theories: the practice of an educative model. Int J Group Psychother 1984; 34:355-368
4. Leszcz M, Yalom ID, Norden M: The value of inpatient group psychotherapy and therapeutic process: patient's perceptions. Int J Group Psychother 1985; 35:177-196
5. Kanas N, Rogers M, Kreth E, et al: The effectiveness of group psychotherapy during the first three weeks of hospitalization: a controlled study. J Nerv Ment Dis 1980; 168:487-492
6. Kline N, Davis J: Group psychotherapy and psychopharmacology, in Comprehensive Group Psychotherapy. Edited by Kaplan HI, Sadock BJ. Baltimore, MD, Williams & Wilkins, 1971
7. O'Brien CP, Hamm KB, Ray BA, et al: Group vs. individual psychotherapy with schizophrenics. Arch Gen Psychiatry 1972; 27:474
8. Kanas N, Barr MA: Homogeneous group therapy for acutely psychotic schizophrenic inpatients. Hosp Community Psychiatry 1983; 34:257-259
9. Barr MA: Homogeneous groups with acutely psychotic schizophrenics. Group 1986; 10:7-12
10. Payn SB: Treating chronic schizophrenic patients. Int J Group Psychother 1974; 24:25
11. Rosen B, Katzoff A, Carrillo C, et al: Clinical effectiveness of 'short' vs. 'long' stay psychiatric hospitalization. Arch Gen Psychiatry 1976; 33:1316-1322

12. Mattes JA, Rosen B, Klein DF: Comparison of the clinical effectiveness of 'short' vs. 'long' stay psychiatric hospitalization, II: results of a three-year post-hospital follow-up. J Nerv Ment Dis 1977; 165:387-394

OUTPATIENT GROUPS   8

Outpatient groups vary dramatically in their clinical situations, goals, and use of various techniques. They may be classified according to the broad aims or thrusts of the group, resulting in four major subdivisions:

1. interpersonal and dynamically oriented groups
2. behaviorally and educationally oriented groups
3. support groups
4. maintenance and rehabilitation groups (Figure 1)

Although this classification serves a heuristic and nosological function, there is a great deal of overlap in goals among the various kinds of outpatient groups. For example, a group for substance abusers that focuses mainly on discrete behavior change and education will also rely heavily on the use of support for its members, and at times will focus exclusively on maintenance and rehabilitation. Or a rehabilitation group for chronic schizophrenics will, at times, make use of gentle interpersonal learning. These limitations notwithstanding, the taxonomy outlined in Figure 1 allows us to understand the broad similarities shared by different kinds of groups, and to turn those similarities into a blueprint for modification of techniques using the three basic steps described in Chapter 7.

Many of these specialized groups are not—strictly speaking—unique to the outpatient setting. Behaviorally and educationally oriented medical subspecialty groups, eating disorders groups, and substance abuse groups also function and flourish on many inpatient units.

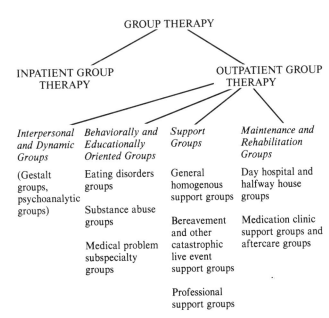

FIGURE 1. **Classification of Outpatient Group Psychotherapy**

■ INTERPERSONAL AND DYNAMIC GROUPS

CLINICAL CONSIDERATIONS AND GOALS

The interpersonal, dynamically oriented group has served as our prototype throughout the text; however, many other forms of group therapy are based on similar principles: psychodrama groups, Gestalt groups, and psychoanalytically oriented groups are all examples of therapy groups which subscribe to the goals of a better understanding of patients' unconscious motivations (dynamics) and interpersonal interactions.

Patients appropriate for such groups are high functioning

and possess a certain degree of insight and motivation to change. Presenting problems or chief complaints are often vague and global, including "unsatisfying relationships with people," "difficulties getting close to others," "depression," "problems with the opposite sex" or "marital strife," "my life is not working," "inability to feel real emotions." The therapist must be able to translate these vague complaints into the language of interpersonal interactions. Often, in fact, the chief complaint is not to be the real problem at all, and it becomes clear to the leader that the person who is complaining of chronic depression and anxiety, for example, actually shows a great deal of hidden rage and passive-aggressive behavior.

The group leader must avoid being drawn into interactions that repeat or reflect the patient's pathology. For example, an articulate, authoritative executive led an unsatisfying romantic life; he only attracted women, he said, who "wanted something from him" or "chased after him." Shortly after he joined a therapy group, he began complaining that things weren't "fast paced" enough and that he wanted to drop out, placing the female therapist and the other members in the unsatisfying role of trying to convince him to stay in the group.

Membership composition in interpersonally and dynamically oriented groups is heterogeneous in terms of underlying problem or pathology, but members are highly similar in ego strength, psychological mindedness, motivation to change, and ability to tolerate interpersonal stimulation. The goals of such groups are not simply relief of the presenting symptom or chief complaint (for, as we have seen, this may not in fact represent the true nature of the underlying problem). These groups propose to effect character change, accompanied by long-lasting change in interpersonal behavior. In order to accomplish this, interpersonal learning will be the single most important therapeutic factor operating in the group.

TASKS AND TECHNIQUES

Most interpersonal and psychoanalytic groups meet once or twice a week for 90 minutes. The optimal membership consists of eight patients, four men and four women, with a male–female co-therapist team. Graduating patients are replaced with new members, but the group is fairly stable since most members, to effect real therapeutic change, remain in the group for one to two years.

Members have the responsibility for introducing topics to open each session, and for self-monitoring the process of the meeting. Continuity between meetings is encouraged by the leaders, through the use of process comments during the sessions, and/or through the use of written summaries between sessions.

The single most important task of the co-therapists is to clarify and interpret the here-and-now. To a certain extent, the exact style and wording of these interpretations is a function of the leaders' ideology and the type of group at hand (Gestalt group, psychodynamic group, etc.). Some leaders prefer to make a summarizing statement at the end of a meeting, while others prefer to intervene whenever there are very strong feelings being expressed, suggesting, for example, that members step back for a moment to try and understand what is happening in the group. Certain therapists wait until they understand the group process thoroughly and then proceed to offer an elaborate and complete interpretation; others intervene much earlier and express hunches, or give tentative and partial explanations.

The most effective means of process interpretation—because it sets the norm for an autonomous and self-monitoring group—is for the therapist to step in and summarize the data at hand, and then to ask members for their explanations. For example: "I'm not sure what's happening today in the group, but I'm aware that Philip and Roger are looking at their watches, and Julie is exchanging glances with Nigel whenever Don is talking. What are your ideas about what's going on?"

The phraseology and the vocabulary of clarifying or interpreting remarks of the therapist will vary according to his or her ideological school. The aim of these remarks, however, is one and the same: to enable the members to understand and assimilate the data arising from the here-and-now interactions of the group. Through the process comments of the leader (and of other members as well), patients are brought to an understanding of their self-presentation, of the impact they have upon others' feelings and opinions, and, consequently, upon their sense of self-worth.

Once patients fully grasp their responsibility for this sequence of events in the group and, by analogy, in life as well, they then grapple with the question, "Am I satisfied with this?" Thera pists who escort their patients through this sequence of events amass great therapeutic leverage and can aid each patient to effect lasting change in his or her interpersonal life.

■ BEHAVIORALLY, COGNITIVELY, AND EDUCATIONALLY ORIENTED GROUPS

Behaviorally, cognitively, and educationally oriented groups all focus on discrete changes in a given pattern of behavior. These groups may or may not make explicit use of the specific techniques of behavioral or cognitive therapy per se, but they share similar goals of promoting change in a patient's maladaptive behavior, and they often show the common features of being structured in nature, closed in membership, and time-limited in duration. Three representative examples are described below: eating disorder groups, substance abuse groups, and medical subspecialty problem groups.

These groups vary in their use of the different therapeutic factors, but all rely heavily on cohesiveness, universality, and the imparting of information, as well as on employing cognitive-behavioral strategies to reduce maladaptive behavior. Some of the groups make limited use of interpersonal learning or self-understanding.

EATING DISORDERS GROUPS

CLINICAL CONSIDERATIONS AND GOALS

Eating disorders groups include groups for people with obesity, anorexia nervosa, or bulimic behavior. Obese patients seeking treatment range from those who wish to lose weight for purely aesthetic reasons, to those who suffer from various medical ailments associated with obesity. They show a varied educational, socioeconomic, and interpersonal background.

Anorexics and bulimics generally consist of young women, often well-educated and of affluent socioeconomic status, and usually described as "high achievers" and "perfectionists." Both anorexics and bulimics have distorted self-images ("I'm fat and unattractive") and show similar concerns about control—and loss of control—over self and food intake. Nonetheless, patients who have restrictive eating behavior should not be mixed in the same group with patients who have bulimia (1, 2). Intense competition can flare up when these two patient populations are treated together. The eating belief systems of anorexics are very rigidly entrenched, and their low weight is a constant reminder to other, nonanorexic patients of their own irrational ideal body weight goals.

Patients with eating disorders—whether morbid obesity, anorexia, or bulimia—keep secret from others their abnormal eating behavior and their obsessive concerns about body image and food. A major goal of group therapy for these patients is to help them share these concerns. Secondly, the group aims to help patients monitor and understand their eating behavior (Table 1).

TASKS AND TECHNIQUES

Eating disorders groups consist of 6 to 12 members and generally meet for a predetermined number of sessions (usually from 8 to 16). Anorexia and bulimia groups are extremely homogeneous with respect to diagnosis, sex, and age group, whereas groups for obese patients are somewhat more heterogeneous in membership. Patients with other major Axis I psychiatric diagnoses are excluded from eating disorders groups.

The therapist must, as of the first session, work vigorously to encourage factual, personal discussions about body image and food intake. Because of the secrecy and shame surrounding their

---

TABLE 1. **General Goals of Eating Disorders Groups**

- Self-disclosure about abnormal eating habits
- Self-disclosure about body image
- Increased understanding about relationship between self-esteem, issues of self-control, body image, and eating habits
- Recognition of cues which provoke abnormal eating behavior
- Recognition of affects associated with abnormal eating behavior
- Education about basic principles of healthy nutrition, exercise, and metabolism
- Identification of interpersonal difficulties related to the eating disorder

abnormal behavior around food, patients with eating disorders experience the process of self-disclosure as a very powerful experience. Self-revelation fosters early group cohesiveness and encourages universality. Open discussions about distorted body image or about abnormal food intake also force members to acknowledge and accept these as essential features of their illness.

Cognitive-behavioral techniques are used in combination with education about the nature of the illness, whether it is obesity, anorexia nervosa, or bingeing-purging. The group therapist teaches patients to look for the cues in their everyday lives which provoke abnormal eating behavior (bingeing on a bag of cookies after a stressful telephone call from mother, for example), and to change their usual thinking patterns about their body and food ("If I weigh more than 100 lbs., I look fat in the hips"). Leaders may also educate members about basic principles of nutrition and metabolism.

Most group programs use self-monitoring techniques to help members understand the factors that influence their eating behavior. Leaders ask members to keep a daily diary and to note the time and amount of food intake, as well as the thoughts and feelings that both trigger and surround eating. Patients learn to identify the situational and psychological factors that lead to bingeing or purging, and they become aware of the cognitions and affects associated with these episodes. The therapist asks each patient to share her findings with the other members of the group, fostering identification and vicarious learning (3).

In a very didactic fashion, the leader helps group members to identify and correct their distorted cognitions associated with eating, self-esteem, and body image ("You believe that your parents are proud of you only because of your looks and your accomplishments"). The therapist also may encourage patients to examine some of their interpersonal difficulties related to these issues through the use of the here-and-now. For example: "Kathy, you've told us you're such a perfectionist, it's hard for you to relax and make friends at school. I wonder if you're not working really hard to be a perfect group member here today."

Leaders specifically advise group members to develop alternative behaviors or strategies whenever they experience the urge to indulge in abnormal eating behavior ("Could you try calling your best friend when you feel blue and just want to binge?"). They offer reinforcement actively whenever a patient describes new, healthier behavior, and they encourage positive feedback from the other group members.

As the end of the group draws near, the therapist must predict the occurrence of relapses and suggest ways of dealing with them; members should be asked to review the new coping mechanisms available to them and strategies to bolster self-esteem when they do relapse. Some leaders encourage post-group socializing as a means of continuing the support system of the group.

SUBSTANCE ABUSE GROUPS

This section will make specific references to treating the alcoholic, although the basic principles are applicable to substance abusers in general.

CLINICAL CONSIDERATIONS AND GOALS

Substance abuse groups are aimed at two general categories of patients: those who are in early recovery and those who are in ongoing recovery. Patients in early recovery have moved into a phase of abstinence, and have accepted the fact that they cannot control their behavior around the use of alcohol. This period of early abstinence is also a period of active dependency, and patients require a great deal of support and structured activity from their group program.

The purpose of early recovery groups is first and foremost to aid patients in maintaining abstinence and in achieving sobriety. This includes supporting patients in staying sober, encouraging AA membership, finding behavioral alternatives to getting intoxicated, and maintaining a treatment plan. The goals of early recovery groups are essentially those of confronting the denial of the alcoholic patient—in other words, of keeping an alcohol focus on any and every problem which arises in the group (Table 2).

As recovery progresses, alcoholic patients begin to experience interdependent, sharing relationships with others, and gain a sense of internal self-reliance as a source of strength and support. "Much of the process of ongoing recovery is the development and fine tuning of the self in relation to a larger whole" (4). At this

TABLE 2. **General Features and Goals of Substance Abuse Groups**

	Early Recovery Groups	Ongoing Recovery Groups	Adult Children of Alcoholics
FEATURES	Members are in first phase of early abstinence	Members are in phase of ongoing abstinence	Members may or may not be substance abusers
	Members are in period of active dependency on group	Members begin to gain a sense of self-reliance	Members use set of characteristic defenses (denial, either/or thinking, need for control, overdeveloped sense of responsibility)
	Members often use a great deal of denial around their substance abuse	Members have overcome their denial around their substance abuse	
GOALS	Support in maintaining sobriety	Maintenance of ongoing abstinence	Confrontation of the ACA's secret: having an alcoholic parent
	Confronting denial about substance abuse	Using interpersonal learning to improve interpersonal relationships	Exploration of effects of growing up with an alcoholic parent
			Helping patients understand their characteristic defenses

point, when substance abusing patients have overcome their denial around the use of substances (usually six to eight months into treatment), they begin to be able to tolerate and learn from interpersonally oriented interactions in the group setting. The goals of ongoing recovery groups thus shift from those of support and an alcohol focus to those of gentle interpersonal learning (Table 2).

The therapist working with alcoholic patients in ongoing recovery must also be aware that many of these patients are the adult children of alcoholics (ACAs). Some groups in alcohol treatment clinics are formed specifically around ACA issues, and include nonalcoholic members who are also ACAs. ACAs share the experience of having grown up in a dysfunctional family, and groups for ACAs are more broad-ranging than those aimed specifically at substance abusers. The primary set of goals for an ACA group relates to helping patients understand their characteristic defensive maneuvers: denial ("My relationship with my wife is wonderful"), either/or thinking ("My daughter is just perfect, but my son is impossible"), a need for control, and an overdeveloped sense of responsibility. Initially, the group will need to confront the single most important issue for each ACA member: uncovering the secret of having an alcoholic parent and of being an adult child of an alcoholic. Later, the group will move on to explore the effects of growing up with such a secret (Table 2).

TASKS AND TECHNIQUES

Oupatient groups for alcoholics and for ACAs take place in a general psychiatry or a specialized drug and alcohol treatment clinic. Patients are referred to the group following detoxification and discharge from an inpatient unit, or following enrollment in an outpatient treatment program; they must participate initially in group therapy that is tailored specifically for the acute stage of recovery. These groups are highly structured and make maximum use of support, and meet daily or at least 3 times a week for 60 to 90 minutes over a 4-week period. Patients may then graduate to early recovery groups that meet once or twice a week over the next 6 to 8 months of recovery.

Therapists leading early recovery groups focus on the substance of abuse (e.g., alcohol), and continuously attempt to identify and examine the problems that members encounter in early abstinence. Patients may introduce topics similar to those discussed in Alcoholics Anonymous (AA) meetings, such as learning to live "just for today," and then feedback around those topics is obtained from all of the members. The group setting provides a complementary structure to the noninteractive mode of AA meetings (4). Concomitant involvement in at least two to three AA meetings weekly is a requirement for patients in early recovery.

The therapist leading early recovery groups must focus continuously on alcohol, challenge patients' use of denial, and help substance abusing patients shift their basic identity and beliefs. Leaders use educational techniques (teaching patients about the physical and psychological effects of alcohol) and behavioral and cognitive interventions (teaching patients to spot the cues that lead them to drink and to come up with alternative strategies).

Some treatment programs prefer to use at least one cotherapist who is a recovering alcoholic. All therapists working with alcoholics should have observed and be familiar with AA meetings; group leaders who wish to make effective confrontations must be familiar with the supportive techniques of AA, including the Twelve Steps, the Twelve Traditions, AA slogans, and the use of a sponsor: "So you're feeling like you're going to slip—Are you doing your twelve steps? Do you have a sponsor?"

Leaders must confront the denial, excuses, justifications, and primitive defenses continuously—such as blaming, projection, sarcastic humor—that occur around the substance use. Although patients will at times want to discuss why they drink, or will want to bring up genetic, developmental, ACA, or co-dependency issues, the therapist in an early recovery group treats this as another defensive maneuver and instead brings the group back to the alcohol focus: "So, you're having a lot of memories about your childhood. How are those memories affecting your drinking behavior now?"

Here-and-now work in the early recovery group is directed toward building positive, constructive bonds between members and toward helping patients to explore and alter behavior that interferes with recovery: for example, their unwillingness to ask for and accept support from others, their arrogance or pride which prevents them from acknowledging their powerlessness over alcohol.

An early recovery group may evolve into an ongoing group, as patients move past the denial phase and can start shifting their focus from alcohol to more interpersonally oriented issues. Ongoing recovery groups permit and even demand an interactive, process-oriented group experience, and they grow increasingly to resemble long-term outpatient groups of nonalcoholic patients. Recognition of differences, here-and-now activation, and interpersonal feedback are now a key part of the group's work, rather than the early, heavy emphasis on support in the early recovery groups.

Individuals in both early and ongoing recovery groups may have slips. Recovery always comes first, and the individual who has slipped must return to a primary focus on abstinence and following the dictates of AA. In a more mature, process-oriented, ongoing recovery group, the group as a whole does not necessarily have to make the shift back to an alcohol focus also, but group members and therapists need to be aware that the drinking compulsion is powerful, and the patient who has slipped will need considerable explicit support from the group.

In ACA groups, or in a mature ongoing recovery group that is confronting ACA issues, the leader must pay particular attention to several other technical concerns. First, he or she must set a very clear external structure, including consistent information and expectations about time and payment issues related to the group. These external limits make the group safe for ACA patients, who are, because of their family background, exquisitely sensitive to threats of disruption, lack of dependability or control, and inconsistency.

Second, therapists involved with ACA groups must use direct support combined with transparency. Because ACA patients grew up in families where denial was the norm, they especially need a group leader who is clear, open, honest, and who consistently works to bring hidden agendas in the group out into the open so that they can be explored gently and safely. Furthermore, because of their chaotic and disruptive upbringing, ACA patients struggle constantly with concerns about what is normal in terms of feelings, reactions, and behavior. Therapists must offer statements such as: "In that situation, I would have felt very hurt and angry." This imparts clear, supportive information about the therapist's emotional experiences.

Leaders in ACA groups must move rapidly and decisively between past experiences and their influence on here-and-now behavior: "Philip, you had to pretend you didn't notice anything when your mother created a scene at parties. I wonder if it's hard for you to acknowledge that Sylvie is really angry here in group today." ACA patients can appear capable, pleasant, compliant, and high achieving, while in fact they are often fragile and brittle.

Under pressure (in the group setting, this translates into a fear of loss of control in the group), they quickly revert back to their familiar defenses (see Table 2).

Leaders of ACA groups, in particular, and of substance abuse groups, in general, must pay particular attention to the countertransference issues that arise in their work. They must avoid overidentification with their hyperresponsible, compliant, self-controlled ACA patients, just as they must avoid acting on their frustration and irritation at the sometimes obsequious or avoidant behavior of their early recovery patients. Supervision or consultation is helpful in aiding the therapist to look at his or her own co-dependency and ACA issues.

MEDICAL SUBSPECIALTY PROBLEM GROUPS

CLINICAL CONSIDERATIONS AND GOALS

Therapy groups for patients in specialized medical settings such as hospitals or specialty clinics are organized around a common disease process (e.g., myocardial infarction, diabetes, multiple sclerosis). They take place in a medical location, such as an intensive care unit, cancer ward, clinic, or hemodialysis unit. They are led by both mental health professionals and other health care workers with specialized training in the patients' illness and treatment. Such groups may follow a fixed format with a set membership for a limited number of sessions, or they may be ongoing in nature, open to members on a drop-in basis, with various topics being discussed as they arise spontaneously in the group. Family members of patients are occasionally included in this group format.

The goals of medical subspecialty problem groups are several: 1) to humanize the treatment environment, 2) to enhance cooperation with medical treatment, 3) to instill hope in their members, and 4) to impart information about specific health problems and about necessary lifestyle changes.

TASKS AND TECHNIQUES

Brief therapy groups in medical settings always begin with the patients' chief concerns: the direct management and impact of their illness. In longer-term, more open-ended groups, such as dialysis or cancer groups, other interpersonally oriented issues may begin to emerge over time and can be addressed in a gentle manner.

Patients with a serious medical illness often learn to express feelings through physical complaints, and the group therapist must be acutely aware of this recurring interpersonal theme. Feelings of anger towards those on whom the patient depends, depression, and feelings of hopelessness all can be translated into a litany of somatic complaints. Medically ill patients also frequently express denial or rebelliousness through treatment non-compliance, or through the sabotaging of treatment plans.

Groups for patients with medical illness do not assume or suggest that the group members' illness is caused by their personality structure or unconscious wishes, drives, or conflicts. Process interpretations are avoided by the group leader. Instead, the leader emphasizes positive coping skills, altruism, and the helpful interactions which occur among group members. Therapists actively encourage patients to be available to each other as sources of information, imitative behavior, and support. Out-group socializing is strongly advocated.

The boundaries of medical subspecialty problem groups are very fluid. Spouses, friends, and other family members can be included regularly or intermittently as a means for them to gain information about the patients' medical problems. The therapist helps patients and their families disabuse themselves of the common fantasy that they are somehow to blame for the illness. Attention is paid to encouraging changes in lifestyle or other habit patterns that might adversely affect the disease, and to emphasizing the fact that the illness is a family affair in which all family members can and should participate.

SUPPORT GROUPS

Support groups are widely encountered both in the self-help movement and in professional contexts. Self-help groups are formed in the lay setting around a particular life problem or life situation and are generally leaderless; their numbers have burgeoned in recent years. Professionally led support groups make use of a trained therapist.

Like medical subspecialty groups, support groups reduce the fear, anxiety, and isolation surrounding a particular situation through the mechanisms of universality and vicarious learning. The development of new coping mechanisms and new strategies for behavior is strongly encouraged.

GENERAL CLINICAL CONSIDERATIONS AND GOALS

Support groups have a homogeneous composition, consisting of members who are united by their struggle with a problem accepted as common to all members. These kinds of groups are organized around shared life problems or symptoms; examples include groups for phobics, persons adjusting to divorce, spouses of Alzheimer's patients, people afflicted with AIDS, the terminally ill, rape victims, and Vietnam veterans.

Support groups are sponsored by many different secular and religious organizations, and the group sessions themselves are held in an extremely wide range of outpatient settings, ranging from church meeting rooms to community centers to clinic conference rooms. Membership number varies widely, depending on the setting and sponsoring organization: a divorce support group held for 3 months in a Jewish community center may have 15 members, while an ongoing biweekly rape crisis group in a women's counseling service may have only 3 or 4 members, with a membership that fluctuates rapidly.

GENERAL TASKS AND TECHNIQUES

Homogeneous support groups are used because emphasizing common struggles is effective therapy for many people. The therapist uses the similarities among group members to foster a sense of universality and cohesion; this helps to combat the feelings of alienation and demoralization that occur when one feels uniquely afflicted in the world.

The underlying assumption from the group members' viewpoint is that one can best be helped by people in the same circumstances, because outsiders do not understand one's unique problems fully. Since members of a support group share so many experiences and can see through each other's facades, they can make demands that each individual come clean about thoughts, feelings, and events that are common to all. A drug addict in a Vietnam veterans' support group, for example, can be challenged vigorously on his choice to "cop out" and "get high" when he experiences the same combat flashbacks that other members experience.

Leaders of support groups encourage members to see themselves as reacting to stress rather than as having intrapsychic or interpersonal conflicts. Not only does the therapist help members to confront what is maladaptive or pathological in each other's behavior—he or she must actively aid patients to be supportive and to find the good in one another. They frequently use a clear agenda, structured exercises, and group problem-solving and advice giving.

As a clinical example, a resident on an AIDS treatment ward reported feeling overwhelmed and depressed by her caseload during a weekly support group meeting. Nursing staff in the group noted that the resident never showed any worry or sadness, and suggested that she begin asking them for help instead of maintaining a facade of confidence. The following week, the resident began to request some help and support whenever she felt anxious about the clinical condition of her patients. When the support group met again, the leader encouraged members to provide positive feedback for the resident's new behavior.

BEREAVEMENT AND OTHER CATASTROPHIC LIFE EVENT GROUPS

CLINICAL CONSIDERATIONS AND GOALS

Support groups for individuals who are recently bereaved, undergoing divorce, or facing a terminal illness are similar in that group members find themselves dealing both with very concrete changes in their normal lifestyle and with complex, abstract, existential issues. Major life events and changes in lifestyle are stressful for the individual on a very day-to-day, practical basis, and the group provides much support for its members at this level. However, members of these kinds of support groups often become involved in discussions about deeper life issues: the meaning of life, the direction their lives have taken, and their personal values and aspirations.

Bereavement is a time of maximum loss and stress; the bereaved (and others facing catastrophic life events) experience the loss of an important defining role, a change in social relationships, and implications for their own mortality. The aim of bereavement support groups is to create a setting in which recent widows and widowers can share their experiences with one another, and in so doing, form a temporary community in which they are deeply understood by peers.

The effects of this are threefold:

1. The group meetings help to combat the social isolation that is so pervasive for the recently bereaved.
2. The discussions provide members, who are experiencing great pain and loss, with a sense of universality.
3. The group provides support for members as they begin to examine the lifestyle changes that lie ahead and as they begin to explore the new contours of their future.

TASKS AND TECHNIQUES

Bereavement groups for widows and widowers are sponsored by community centers, religious organizations, and private, non-profit self-help organizations. Many run for a limited number of sessions (8 to 12) with a closed membership, but some are ongoing and open in nature.

Groups for those facing catastrophic life events, such as bereavement, are generally highly successful. Members grow deeply engaged; trust, cohesion and self-disclosure are high; meetings are often powerful, and attendance excellent. Recent research further attests to the efficacy of spousal bereavement groups: At one year follow-up, widows and widowers who have high initial levels of distress are significantly helped by an eight-session group experience held six months after bereavement, as compared to a no-group control population (6).

Leaders must establish norms for a safe and supportive group, encourage gentle process review, and make here-and-now interventions when appropriate, tailoring them to specific issues of bereavement and personal change as they surface in the group. For example, when Mary, an orderly and shy woman who had always subordinated herself to her boisterous husband, expressed concern about taking too much time in the spousal bereavement group when she spoke, the therapist focused on her self-abnegation by exploring her feeling of having taken up too much time:

"How do the other members view that? What are the *shoulds* for behavior in this group? Where did they come from?"

An intervention which focuses on "shoulds"—personal or perceived societal behavioral expectations—is particularly relevant for catastrophic life event groups. Members inevitably find it helpful to reflect on the yoke of "shoulds" they carry around: One should grieve for a whole year, one should quickly give away all of the spouse's belongings, one should not be alone during the weekend, or one should not develop a new sexual relationship for some prescribed period of time.

Because loss is such a major issue for members of bereavement groups, the leader's role as timekeeper is very important. In time-limited groups, therapists may prod group members with the powerful tool of anticipated regret: "There are only four more meetings left. If the group were to end now, what would you regret not having shared with us?"

Specific structured exercises, such as asking members to bring in wedding photographs, are helpful in eliciting new material for discussion or in encouraging self-disclosure. In general, therapists must be very attentive to the timing of structured exercises lest they hamper the more spontaneous interactions and discussions surfacing in the bereavement group (7).

Therapists must be knowledgable about the issues and themes that preoccupy bereaved spouses (or others facing catastrophic life events) in order to facilitate the emergence and discussion of these themes in the group setting. The most important of these for the bereaved are the themes of change, time and ritual, new relationships, and existential issues (Table 3). Two themes are especially rich in content for bereaved spouses and share a certain interrelatedness: the theme of change (the transition from "we" to "I"), and the existential theme of responsibility for oneself and one's own life. Over the course of bereavement groups, leaders must be aware that members struggle with complex questions of growth, identity, and responsibility for the future.

PROFESSIONAL SUPPORT GROUPS

CLINICAL CONSIDERATIONS AND GOALS

Professional support groups are designed to help profes-

TABLE 3. Major Themes in Bereavement Support Groups

Change:	How does one make the transition from "We" to "I"?
	Who am I?
	What gives me my sense of myself, of my own identity?
Time and ritual:	How long should I grieve?
	Why are rituals so helpful?
New relationships:	How long before I can start new love relationships?
	Is new love a betrayal of the deceased spouse?
Existential issues:	I've worked hard, led a good life. Why is fate so unjust?
	What have I learned about my own mortality?
	How can I live the life remaining to me to the fullest?
	My meaning in life was to be a wife (husband). How can I find meaning now? No one cares if I'm alive or dead. I'm alone and I'm free.

sionals deal with highly stressful working environments, such as occur on intensive care units (ICUs), in residency training programs, on wards with patients suffering from AIDS, and occasionally in certain corporate settings. Many work-related complaints and concerns about professional "burn-out" surface in these kinds of groups. Common examples include:

1. frustration over excessive work loads and inadequate staffing or administrative support
2. anger at the distribution of actual or perceived power
3. feelings of insecurity and inadequacy stemming from enormous professional responsibilities and a constant pressure to perform under stress
4. clashes in interpersonal style with co-workers

Those in helping professions and those working in clinical settings carry the additional burden of facing continuous issues of loss, chronicity, disfigurement, and death.

Professional support groups are organized occasionally in

response to a particular crisis or catastrophe, such as when the administrative clinicians managing an acute psychiatric service arrange a staff retreat to deal with management changes. Group meetings may continue on a weekly or monthly basis, or as part of an annual workshop or retreat. Responsibility for organizing support groups usually lies with administrators or management level individuals, who may then choose to have an outside consultant lead or facilitate the group.

The general goal of professional support groups is to increase communication about work-related issues and to reduce unnecessary emotional tension in the workplace. The interaction of the needs of the individual versus the needs of the professional organization or structure (for example, staff versus client needs in a substance abuse clinic) is generally one of the most powerful underlying themes in the group. Sessions may also be strictly problem-oriented, and may have specific aims such as teaching staff how to cope with an abusive patient, helping members to develop strategies to manage time more effectively, or instructing individuals in relaxation exercises.

TASKS AND TECHNIQUES

The therapist leading a professional support group attempts to foster an open, collegial atmosphere in which common problems are examined together, rather than an analytic atmosphere that encourages deep scrutiny of intrapsychic conflict. Issues stemming from outside the workplace are avoided at first, but the impact of personal life events, such as marriages, divorces, motherhood, maternity leave, and the like, eventually surface and need to be examined insofar as they affect professional performance.

Once the individuals organizing the support group have decided upon its format (for example, the human resources department of a small software company asks a therapist to lead six "problem-solving" meetings with all management level employees)—the leader must begin to structure the sessions. It is important, especially in early meetings, that the group not focus too strongly on the behavior or problem of any one group member. Members must seek instead to find problems common to all individuals in the group. Groups often strive to identify a "patient"—it provides an engaging topic and catalyzes early sessions; soon, however, it leads to scapegoating and is counterproductive.

Instead, the therapist must encourage altruism and advice-giving by asking more experienced members to share with others the means by which they cope with the stresses of the working environment and to describe the ongoing problems they still find difficult to master. If the group is an angry one, then it is best to have members systematically and openly identify all of their major stresses and frustrations, rather than to have such feelings leak out indirectly and obliquely in the group ("These meeting times are really interfering with my department's deadlines"). The therapist will need to titrate the expression of conflict and hostile feelings very carefully. Too early and too forceful expressions of direct anger or confrontation is extremely threatening to group cohesion.

Various professional support groups vary in their overall ability to integrate here-and-now interactions. A group for psychiatry residents, for example, will certainly be able to benefit from here-and-now activation and process illumination. An ICU support group for nurses who are continuously working on the front lines may not find these same interventions helpful; for one thing, members may have a greater investment in dealing with job-related stress and at first may not be interested in confronting interpersonal staff tensions. Only later, after the development of positive feelings and mutual interdependence, can interpersonal tensions and deficiencies in performance be explored gently and supportively.

Professionals in demanding careers at times feel powerful, competent, and effective—and at other times feel like impostors and feel impotent and ineffectual. A sense of effectiveness can be enhanced by encouraging members to identify and examine the specific issues that threaten their feelings of competence. They may also be encouraged to come to a consensus around a particular challenge; for example, members of a psychology internship will feel an increased sense of power when they act as a group to confront an administrative decision affecting their training. At the same time, the leader of a professional support group must be careful to avoid promoting behavior that simply represents acting out by the group around a volatile issue, or of setting up such a charged situation in the group that splitting and subgrouping become inevitable.

"Burn-out" is a particularly important theme in groups of

busy professionals. Members describe being unable to forget the job when away from work, or losing the capacity for pleasure, play, or true relaxation. Some are workaholics, or anhedonic, or chronically unhappy with their workplace. Many are substance abusers. Group therapists can employ and teach tension-reducing physical or psychological techniques, such as relaxation exercises, guided imagery, and self-hypnosis. These techniques are especially important during weekend retreats or lengthy workshops.

Professional support groups are best held over a finite number of sessions or a finite time frame. This emphasizes that group members are basically healthy, have intact abilities to cope and to problem-solve, and are not in need of formal treatment. These kinds of support groups underline the strength and competency of professionals who are encouraged to see themselves as reacting to the environmental pressures of the workplace. Keeping professional support groups time-limited, but part of a repetitive, continuing pattern that is scheduled and anticipated in advance (such as an annual staff retreat), is helpful. This format helps to integrate new members and allows for periodic reexamination of professional stressors, coping skills, and interpersonal interactions in the workplace.

■ MAINTENANCE AND REHABILITATION GROUPS

Maintenance and rehabilitation groups aim to treat patients with chronic mental illness or chronic behavioral problems in various outpatient settings. Many of the same general principles discussed in the section on chronic inpatient groups in Chapter 7 apply to this population.

DAY HOSPITAL AND RESIDENTIAL TREATMENT GROUPS

Day hospitals and halfway houses serve two roles: They provide patients recently discharged from the hospital with a transitional living situation, and they provide an ongoing stable and structured treatment setting for patients who might otherwise require hospitalization.

CLINICAL CONSIDERATIONS AND GOALS

In day hospitals and halfway houses, patients either spend the day or reside in a facility that provides a comprehensive, structured treatment program with scheduled duties and activities. Programs make use of occupational therapy, leisure pursuits, exercise and outings, and group psychotherapy. Different treatment programs deal with very different clinical populations. Some day hospitals and halfway houses work with a mixed population of patients with chronic psychotic illness plus patients with a melange of other psychiatric diagnoses. Other day treatment programs or residential treatment programs exclude patients who require psychotropic medication, or who have a history of psychosis. In general, patients who are a severe behavioral challenge, who are actively suicidal, or who are acutely psychotic are not suitable for these kinds of programs.

The overall goal in day hospitals and halfway houses is to model real life, and to emphasize real tasks. Patients in these programs usually work part-time on a regular basis, either at a paying job, at volunteer work, or in various practical tasks around the place of residence. Patients' reactions to and ways of dealing with these structured work activities are important material to be examined in group meetings.

Day hospitals and residential treatment programs use three different kinds of groups with three different sets of goals in their treatment programs:

1. Patients' interpersonal strategies are examined in small groups
2. Life-like situations focused on cooperation and responsibility are created in task-oriented or chore group settings, such as community meetings
3. Social skills learning occurs in controlled social groups.

In addition, day hospital and residential treatment programs are built around three other important features:

1. specific rules for permissible conduct
2. an elected governing body made up of patients from the treatment program

3. set agendas for at least some of the group meetings, such as the daily community meetings

The manner in which different patients react to the set rules and regulations, for example, or participate in self-government, quickly reveals aspects of their personality and psychopathology that can be explored further in group work (8). The overall goal for the groups is to achieve rehabilitation and support (Table 4).

TASKS AND TECHNIQUES

Day hospitals and residential programs have daily community meetings, in which all patients participate, as well as smaller treatment groups that meet from three to six times a week. Community meetings are usually run by the patient-elected governing body and have set agendas (distributing chores, solving general complaints, planning outings). Treatment groups consist of four to eight patients meeting regularly with one or two therapists to focus on specific interpersonal or social skills issues.

Because the underlying precept of the treatment program is to provide safe, helpful structure for patients, part of the task of the group work is to support and reinforce the structure of the program; for example, by examining tensions among patients or among patients and staff. Unlike work in a prototypic interaction group, established norms for behavior (or group members' responsibility for changing norms) cannot be questioned in the day hospital or residential treatment group. On the contrary, the patients' reactions to the established norms and expectations for behavior are important therapeutic information and part of the material that gets explored in the group work.

TABLE 4. **Goals for Day Hospital and Residential Treatment Groups**

- Restitution of appropriate level of psychological functioning

- Correction of maladaptive interpersonal strategies

- Improvement of patients' functioning in structured, task-oriented environment

- Support for patient's efforts to develop new skills and coping mechanisms in social and work settings

There must be clear expectations for punctual attendance and for honest communication in meetings. Group leaders must actively discourage divisive subgrouping or scapegoating, and must help members learn that their progress is intimately related to the progress of others. The tight-knit system of committee structures, daily activities, and group sessions puts patients in the position of co-responsibility for their own and others' welfare. The therapist encourages patients to be active in several various roles, and in this way to gain greater mastery over their lives and to develop new interpersonal patterns.

MEDICATION CLINIC GROUPS AND CHRONIC AFTERCARE GROUPS

CLINICAL CONSIDERATIONS AND GOALS

Medication clinic groups and chronic aftercare groups are targeted for the chronic mentally ill and have several goals: education about psychotropic medications, discussion of medication side effects, enhancement of compliance with outpatient treatment planning, and the provision of support and socialization (9–11).

Groups typically meet from once a week to once every two weeks, and at times as infrequently as once a month. They are held at the patient's outpatient clinic as part of a medication review appointment or as part of routine scheduled follow-up. They may be held prior to or following the patient's regular meeting with his or her caseworker or psychiatrist; at times, they replace the individual meeting. Groups are occasionally built around a specific issue (current events, social skills) or around a specific medication (for example, a lithium group). The majority of patients attending medication clinic groups have a chronic psychotic illness and are treated with a variety of long-term antipsychotic medications.

TASKS AND TECHNIQUES

Although the major principles of group work with this population are similar to those employed in groups for lower-functioning acute inpatients and for chronic inpatients, there are four specific concerns that are characteristic of medication clinic groups and chronic aftercare groups.

The first of these is education about psychotropic medication and medication effects. Although some didactic teaching can and should come from the group leader, the leader should also encourage advice-giving among patients over issues of target symptoms and side effects. Patients often find this an engaging topic and avidly compare notes, thus fostering safe, nonprovocative interpersonal interchange.

Second, most patients with a chronic psychotic illness have had auditory hallucinations, have felt paranoid, or have had periods of disorganized and confused thinking. These symptoms provide patients in the group with a common topic for discussion, and members can disconfirm each other's unusual experiences. For example, a patient may report he is troubled by voices talking directly to him from the television; less psychotic members can reassure him that they do not hear the same voices, and that while the experience may seem real, the voices are not real. The therapist then encourages a general discussion of useful strategies for coping with hallucinations. Patients can share the various techniques they have found helpful for coping with troublesome symptoms, such as avoiding stressful situations, taking an as needed medication dose, listening to music, talking to a friend, or engaging in a hobby. In like manner, patients with paranoid ideation can disconfirm their suspicions by learning to ask group members, in a nonconfrontational manner, if their fears are true.

Many chronic psychiatric patients, because of their lack of trust and poor interpersonal skills, lead lonely, isolated lives. Consequently, a third concern of the medication clinic group or the chronic aftercare group is the improvement of social skills. The therapist must direct patients to try new ways of communicating: "Wendy, could you tell us what it was like to go to your sister's birthday party?" Or: "Wendy, Terry is worried about the upcoming family reunion he has to go to—what are some of the ways you have found to cope with your family?"

Fourth, allowing patients to express their feelings over the stigma and sequelae of their illness can also lead to productive meetings. Patients benefit from discussions concerning their loneliness, their sense of alienation, and their despair about ever getting better, discussions which at times take an existential bent. The group leader will need to be empathic, without resorting to either condescension or exaggerated optimism: "The world seems very unfair when you think about having to live with a chronic illness." Although anger discussed as a general issue, such as anger at life or fate, or anger referred to people or events outside of the group may be tolerated, anger expressed among group members must be managed decisively by the therapist and the topic should be changed diplomatically.

The encouragement and feedback that patients receive from their peers in the group augments compliance with medications and treatment planning, and decreases clinic drop-outs far more effectively than follow-up using a one-to-one format. Education, support, safety, and continuity are the mainstays of medication clinic groups; when run successfully, they go far in helping patients to remain in treatment and to decrease episodes of rehospitalization (10, 11).

■ REFERENCES

1. Inbody DR, Ellis JJ: Group therapy with anorexic and bulimic patients: implications for therapeutic intervention. Am J Psychother 1985; 39:411-420
2. Mackenzie KR, Livesley WJ, Coleman M, et al: Short-term group psychotherapy for bulimia nervosa. Psychiatric Annals 1986; 16:699-708
3. Schneider JA, Agras WS: A cognitive-behavioral group treatment of bulimia. Br J Psychiatry 1985; 146:66-69
4. Brown: Treating the Alcoholic: A Developmental Model of Recovery. New York, Wiley, 1985
5. Weiner MF: Homogeneous groups, in Psychiatry Update: American Psychiatric Association Annual Review, Volume 5. Edited by Frances AJ, Hales RE. Washington, DC, American Psychiatric Press, 1986
6. Lieberman M, Yalom ID: Short-term bereavement groups: a controlled study. Manuscript in preparation
7. Yalom ID, Vinogradov S: Bereavement groups: techniques and themes. Int J Group Psychother
8. Lazerson JS: Intergrated psychotherapy at the Day House. Psychiatric Annals 1986; 16:709-714
9. Payn SB: Group methods in the pharmacotherapy of chronic psychotic patients. Psychiatr Q 1965; 39:258
10. Herz MI, Spitzer RL, Gibbon M, et al: Individual vs. group aftercare treatment. Am J Psychiatry 1974; 131:808
11. Masnik R, Olarte SW, Rosen A: Coffee groups: a nine-year follow-up study. Am J Psychiatry 1980; 137:91-93

9 CONCLUSION

Group psychotherapy is employed in a vast number of clinical settings with a proven degree of effectiveness. It makes use of various therapeutic factors or mechanisms of change, many of them unique to group psychotherapy. Some of these therapeutic factors—such as universality, altruism, catharsis, and the imparting of information—are widely encountered in many different kinds of groups, whereas the potent but often misunderstood factor of interpersonal learning requires a skilled and experienced therapist working in a specialized interactional setting. Various constellations of these therapeutic factors operate in different types of groups at different times.

All clinicians should be familiar with the specific techniques and interventions used in group psychotherapy; these include working in the here-and-now, therapist transparency, and the use of various procedural aids. Fundamental techniques can be modified to suit any specialized group setting, from the acute inpatient group to the symptom-oriented outpatient group. Indeed, the power of group therapy lies in its adaptability: It is a flexible and efficient mode of psychotherapy that can accommodate a wide range of settings, goals, and patients.

INDEX

166